THE ONES THAT BIT ME!

MARCUS TAYLOR

THE ONES THAT BIT ME!

CAMELS, COWS & OTHER YOUNG-VET STORIES

MASSEY UNIVERSITY PRESS

AUTHOR'S NOTE

The names of people and some locations have been altered, and in rare instances the details of different cases have been merged to protect the privacy of those involved. However, the details and the events described remain as the author recalls them.

This book is dedicated to my sister, who encouraged me to start it, and to my wife, whose love and support allowed me to finish it.

CONTENTS

PREFACE

IT ALL BEGAN WITH A TURKEY. We stood eye-to-eye, locked in a toddler–bird standoff. I was three years old, so we were of equal intelligence, but the turkey had an edge. I wanted to flick his gobbley little neck and make it wobble. He wanted me to go away. I toddled towards him. He raised his head, gaining a height advantage but exposing his flappy neck, the object of my wonder. I made my move but before my hand had gone an inch he struck. *TAP! TAP! TAP!* Three sharp pecks to the forehead, and I toppled onto my backside, screaming in outrage. A decisive defeat.

On a family trip to Australia a few years later, I plucked a blue-green, glass-eyed lizard from a rock and clasped it in my hand. With primal speed, the agitated reptile twisted in my hands, clamping her jaws onto my finger. I ran shrieking to my parents, the lizard still dangling from my hand.

Later that year, back home in New Zealand, I tangled with a colossal longfin eel, shimmering and black, monstrous yet elegant. She must have been 80 years old. She twisted at the river's edge, tangled among dozens of other eels looking for food. I leaned down and put my hand in the water. One hungry chomp later and my blood filled the stream, sending the swarming eels into a frenzy.

The next year, we took our annual holiday at a deep-green lake nestled between mountains on the West Coast.

My fingers were dusted with sugary powder after a leisurely marshmallow-toasting session when a dragonfly so large that he belonged in *King Kong* choppered down to land on my hand. I was enchanted by his black-and-yellow colouring and bulbous eyes. I held still, revelling in my apparent abilities as an animal-whisperer. Here I was in a remote wilderness, attracting beautiful creatures. The small dragon crept his way towards my fingertips, pausing at the sugar. That's it: explore, friend. When his jaws locked down, piercing skin and flesh, my scream echoed across the lake . . .

By the time I had graduated from veterinary school at the age of 23, a sheep, a cow, a hawk, innumerable dogs, cats, parrots and even a territorial fish had locked their mandibles onto my flesh. Every bite only intrigued me further. The wonderful creatures with which we share this planet have never stopped filling me with awe, and it is for them that I've written this book about my adventures as a vet.

CHAPTER ONE

WRESTLING THE MOON COW

I KICKED OFF MY GUMBOOTS and pushed the front door open with my elbow, not wanting to dirty the handle. My day in the trenches had left me covered in every manner of excreta; my aroma arrived home before I did. The main female in my life came racing to meet me in the hallway, fascinated and ready to spend as long as I'd allow her sniffing my sleeves, arms and face. I was a house cat's dream. Unfortunately, my human roommates were not as thrilled.

Here was my dilemma: I was on call. If I didn't shower, chances were I wouldn't be called out and I'd have stayed stinky for no reason. But, invariably, every time I showered when I was on call — *Ding!* — the ominous toll of my work phone sounded.

The evening of the 'moon-cow wrestling' would be one of those unfortunate occasions.

Ding!

> Cow down in paddock,
> difficulty calving.

Just from the text, I knew I was in for a tough night. The cow was in distress — and she was also not on her feet. When a pregnant cow is lying down, there is less space to work with inside the uterus, making it harder to extricate the calf, meaning I'd have to work either sitting or lying on the ground, in knee-deep mud. So it was with some apprehension that I climbed into my truck, my hair dripping, and smelling like a soap shop.

Soon the wide roads of Canterbury were disappearing behind me as the spring sun dipped behind the Southern Alps. The contrast to my life of two weeks earlier was stark. Then, I had been wandering the streets of Lisbon, drinking red wine with a gorgeous woman named Lila whose sand-blonde hair fell in loose curls, framing her wide blue eyes. Chasing her had felt like trying to catch a speck of dust floating in a beam of light. Every time I got close, she danced away. I sighed and hoped the calf wouldn't be as tricky to pin down.

By the time I pulled into the hedge-rimmed paddock the sun had finished its lazy fall behind the mountains. Twilight was setting in. A stubby older chap in mud-stained overalls waved me over. His grey hair was short and there was stubble on his weathered cheeks. There are many like him in New Zealand — but none the same — archetypal hard-working Kiwis who walk their paddocks at all hours, making sure their animals are safe, and who grind away at the seemingly endless list of tasks on the farm before finally heading home to dinner and the fireplace.

The farmer looked troubled and seemed jumpy as he

made his way over to my truck, confirming my fears that this might not be a run-of-the-mill call-out.

'Sheza-goer. She'll go ya, shehwill!' His rapid-fire sentences blended words into a language of their own.

'Dahryt?' I answered, grateful that I'd grown up close enough to farm gates to pick up an ear for this unique dialect.

'Yep, shezhaddacrackahme, o'll tell ya. A reeeal goer,' he warned.

Translation: She attacked me, so look out.

The farmer's eyes were wide, and there was a tremor in his voice. Given his obvious years of farming experience, this anxiety surprised me.

I turned my attention to the cow. Her head was turned back in our direction, and she was glaring at us. Her eyes were wild, and her head twitched. Ketosis. A condition that occurs when an animal's blood sugar is very low, it can send cattle into a hyperactive, aggressive frenzy. Prolonged labour, like the kind this cow was experiencing, is a common cause.

Even from where I was standing, I could see the nose of her partially born calf sticking out of her back end, and it didn't look like it was moving in a hurry. I paused to consider my options. None of them looked great.

To my astonishment, I realised my companion was already creeping like a midnight assassin towards the nervous cow. I hadn't even had time to grab my rope. Left with little choice, I joined him, planning to time my dash along with his. We would jump on her head and immobilise her before she could get to her feet and charge us. I moved towards the cow, creeping a little faster to catch up with the farmer. Again, I underestimated his eagerness. Within seconds, he had dashed ahead of me and leapt onto the cow with full gusto.

'HEAWEGO!' he bellowed.

The panicked cow thrashed her head from side to side as he landed on her muscular neck. Head-to-head the two struggled before she managed to toss him off, flailing like a doll. He pounced back. Most people would have considered surrendering at this point, but this warrior had 60 years' worth of farmer strength and resilience to call on. I ran as fast as I could towards the manic scene. He held on tight, and seconds later I joined the fray.

'GEDDER!' he cried, as I landed half on him and half on the cow.

Together we grappled her head around, so her nose was next to her side. I held her head tight until the farmer got a good grip. Eventually, she huffed and let her head settle on the cool grass. Once things calmed, I slid from her shoulders to get my calving equipment. Surrounding us, a semicircle of curious, liquid-eyed cattle held their heads low, sniffing in our direction. More cows standing behind them craned their necks, bearing witness to the scene.

Now that the farmer had the distressed cow in hand, I could return to the truck to get the equipment I needed. Rummaging around, I found my ropes and swung them around my arm. I then grabbed a 2-metre-long narrow steel device called a calving jack, which uses a ratchet system to apply traction to a calf when it is stuck. Next, my vet's box of tricks. It was only then, reaching back in the rapidly vanishing light, that I realised I'd forgotten the last piece of essential equipment: a headlamp. Calving a cow is tricky enough without doing it in the dark.

'I'll need you to hold her still while I pull the truck up so we have some light,' I told the farmer.

By now, the farmer was perched comfortably on his steed. He looked at the rising full moon on the horizon.

'Yull have light frum the moon!' he crowed.

I pondered this for a moment, then agreed. The idea of calving by moonlight was intriguing after all.

I made my way back over and put my gear down. The cow had relaxed a little, and was now obligingly lying on her side. From his warm cow seat the farmer was gazing out at the final flare of golden light vanishing behind the mountains; he'd relaxed, too, it seemed.

I gave the cow an epidural, carefully inserting a long needle between the vertebrae at the base of her tail. Next, I cleaned her back end, then washed my hands and forearms. I rubbed thick orange lube on my arms, and then checked her inside. I was met with a familiar warmth, and my cold fingers thawed a little. The calf was wedged with its nose just protruding from its mother's vulva. One of its front legs was coming hoof-forward, with the elbow stuck back beside its chest. The other leg was still tucked all the way back and well out of reach.

I put my fingers in the calf's mouth and it moved its tongue, confirmation that it was still alive. A correctly presenting calf comes out like Superman, taking its first heroic dive into the world — a serious drop for a newborn calf from a standing cow's backside. If they are one of the luckier ones, the cow will give birth lying on her side. It always baffled me how the little calves managed to avoid injury, plonking down onto the grass from such a height.

But this calf wasn't going anywhere in its current position. I ran a clear rubber tube into the mother's birth canal and positioned it over the calf, then pumped lube around it.

I started Plan A. Placing my hand on the calf's forehead, I tried to push it back into the cow. The calf didn't budge. I changed tactics and tried sliding my hand past the calf's neck, hoping I could get its malpresenting leg up, but the leg was on the side of the cow that lay on the ground. All her weight was crushing my hand, and I grunted in pain as I tried to push through. The farmer turned to watch me and raised an eyebrow. I was thwarted. Damn. I settled with extending the calf's leg that was already pointed forward all the way out, so that it stuck out of the cow's back end alongside its head.

Time for Plan B. We needed to roll the cow onto her other side so that I had more space to free the leg. We sat her up on her haunches, and of course she tried to stand and throw us once more.

'Watchit! She'll go ya!' the farmer cried for a second time.

We wrestled with her swinging neck and concrete-hard head. Finally, we pulled her head around again, this time the other way. Together, we planted our shoulders, one just above the armpit and the other on her hips, and drove with our legs, heaving her over onto her other side. It's no wonder New Zealand has so much success in rugby: half the nation spends its time tackling and scrummaging livestock.

Around us silver moonlight reflected off the watchful eyes of the other curious cattle. The paddock and surrounding trees had transformed into a magical grey-scape under the glow of the moon.

After washing my hands again, I reached back in. To my disappointment, I still couldn't get past the calf's shoulder to reach the misplaced leg. The cow's birth canal was too narrow. Time for Plan C: gentle traction.

I wouldn't normally pull a calf out with one leg back, but it was my last option and worth a try. I pumped even more lube over the calf and looped my rope around the front leg, just above the calf's carpal joint, which is the equivalent of a human's wrist. I then made a second loop just below its carpus to reduce the pressure from the pull. Next, with a separate rope, I made a bigger loop that I slipped over the calf's head, making sure it went all the way behind its ears and pulled tight in its mouth. Then I picked up my calving jack.

The calving jack is used by first bracing it against the cow's back end. A long metal bar extends about 2 metres back from the brace. On the metal bar is a ratchet system from which you can attach ropes. Now, I know what you might be thinking. This barbaric chap is about to pull the head off the poor wee thing! I petition for a delay in your assessment. Would I accost you with such a tale so early in the piece?

Newborn calves are very different to newborn babies. Their bones, including their skulls and jaws, are developed and strong. They are designed to be on their feet and running within the hour — the alternative is to be lion's tucker. Well, at least it was where they originally came from; there isn't as much as a toothed goose to pose a threat to anything larger than a well-fed guinea pig here in Kiwiland. Although a great deal of care is still required, due to this handy design you can put more traction on a calf than you might think.

I placed the calving jack brace against the cow's back end, then wrapped the ropes around the hooks on the ratchet. Slowly, I increased the tension on the ropes by working the ratchet.

The farmer peered over the cow's back as I worked. I gradually added tension and angled the device so that it was pulling the calf in a downward direction as well as out. With each pull, the calf inched from the cow. An eye appeared, then an ear, then a shoulder . . . until, all at once, the little female calf came rushing out, slithering from her mother, shiny and slippery in her foetal membranes. She made a wet splat as she landed on the grass. I removed the ropes and cleared her nose.

All my attention was now on the calf as I pulled mucous

from her nose and mouth, then vigorously rubbed her over the ribs. I heaved her up off the ground to let the last of the birth fluids drain from her nose and mouth. My back strained as I lifted her by the waist, gently swinging her from side to side, allowing gravity to do the work. Slimy mucous glinted in the moonlight as it ran from her nose and pooled on the grass. Still, she lay limp in my arms. Despite my efforts, she wouldn't breathe. Had I pulled too hard? Had I taken too long?

I rubbed the calf's slimy back firmly with one arm, then slapped the side of her chest to stimulate her. I put my fingers in her nose and pinched between her nostrils.

Wake up! My muscles screamed as I held the heavy, limp calf in the air.

Then, a cough. She took her first breath. Slow, wet and ragged as it was, there was life. Relief rolled over me as I laid her on the grass in a dog's sitting position so she could breathe more easily. Once she was breathing well, I turned my attention back to the cow. I put my hand in to check for a twin or for any damage to the uterus. She felt fine, and the farmer, still roosted on her side, chirped his satisfaction.

I injected her with oxytocin to help close the uterus, along with antibiotics, pain relief and a calcium-glucose mix. I had one final wrestle with her to get some more glucose, an added measure against ketosis, into her mouth. Before I'd finished, she was clambering to her feet. The dismounted farmer made a dash for it, anticipating a vengeful charge that never came.

Our ever-faithful bovine observers let out a silent cheer

for me and my new friends. Exhausted but triumphant, I made my way back to the truck.

As I filled out the paperwork, my new comrade told me a story that explained his somewhat surprising degree of nervousness, given his obvious years of farming experience. A few years back he had been bowled down and savagely gored by a bull that had mashed him into the ground and smashed his ribs. Sharp hooves had stomped him again and again, pummelling him into the dirt, breaking skin and cracking bones. The bull was rearing up and thumping down with his full weight, crushing the poor man's crumpled body.

Just as he had given up hope of surviving the onslaught, his son came hurtling into the paddock, running at the beast with a stick in his hand. He'd saved his father's life. The farmer had been nervy around cattle ever since. I viewed his earlier leap onto the cow's head with a new sense of awe as he finished his tale.

It was with some satisfaction that I noticed the cow sniffing and then licking her calf. I said my goodbyes to the gentleman and the four-legged onlookers and loaded the last of my things back into the truck. The hot steam from my shower earlier that evening had been replaced with sweat, mud and foetal fluids, but I drove home smiling, the image of the stocky man flying through the air fresh in my mind. What an absolute legend.

CHAPTER TWO

VET SCHOOL

Ten years earlier . . .

THE CAR SLOWED TO A STOP. The headlights lit the outside of a run-down flat. I could hear shouting and music coming from the backyard. Beside me in the back seat, Pepper casually adjusted the collar on her overalls.

Olive turned around from the driver's seat. 'Are you sure you want to do this?' she asked, raising her eyebrows. 'It would be better to wait until the first wave of the other first-years goes in: the first ones in always get it the worst . . .'

Becca chuckled beside her in the front. 'I'm going to wait with Olive. The cannon fodder can go first.' She shooed us from the car like pesky chooks.

Pepper and I clambered out into the cool winter's night. At the side of the house, a huge ram's skull was being lowered from a tree by a rope. Pepper and I were both dressed in dark-green overalls, having been warned by the older students to be prepared for the worst.

The four of us had completed our entry papers in

Auckland, studying together almost every day. The stress of competing with hundreds of other students for a few coveted spots in the school had bonded us like troopers. About 40 of us were applying from Auckland. The lecturers had said that usually only two or three students get through from the Auckland group. This year, it was we four. It certainly helped that Olive already had an engineering degree, and Pepper and Becca had both been part-way through med school when they'd decided to make the jump to veterinary medicine. I was the limpet that had latched on and made friends with the right people.

That night, it was possible we were the only ones from our class brave enough or stupid enough to turn up. We were first-years. And we were to be initiated into vet school.

'I'll go first,' I announced as we approached the open front door. 'Stay close!'

Pepper shoved me aside. 'We both know you're a lightweight Christian schoolboy who is going to tip over at the first whiff of something stronger than a ginger beer. I'll go first.'

'Damn, Pepper.' I feigned indignation. 'And I thought the terrorising happened inside.'

She strode ahead, flung the door open and was gone. Without anyone to masquerade for, my confidence fell away. I approached the open door and edged inside. Clammy hands grabbed me and pulled me to one side. I felt cold steel as a drench gun nozzle was shoved between my teeth. The device, reserved for sheep, had a new and noble role that night. First-years. A laughing girl squeezed the trigger and a jet of burning liquid hit the back of my throat. I swallowed like an obliging lamb, then looked for Pepper. She had vanished.

'Baaaaaah!' the lass cried into my ear. 'Yeah! That's the one.' She laughed again, her curly ginger hair bobbing. 'Wait here,' she ordered, then headed through a door, shutting it behind her.

Chanting came from the next room, and, before I had time to recover, the girl returned and shoved me through the door. I hit a wall of musky heat — the kind of wet warmth that can only be generated by hundreds of bodies crammed together in a small space. I caught a glimpse of Pepper disappearing out another door. Was that blood on her face? Was she hurt? She gave me a wink and waved as she sauntered off.

People were crowding in, red-faced and chattering. I was pushed into the centre of the room and a circle formed around me. The group hushed as a tall, sharp-featured man stepped forward to speak; the rabble had a leader.

'From the skull he shall drink!' he announced.

A deep chant of 'Ohu!' boomed from the students. Then silence.

'The knowledge of the ram shall flow to you!' the leader continued.

'Ohu!' the crowd bellowed, their feet falling into a unified stomp.

'It is better to behold than to tame!' he pronounced to the ceiling.

'Ohu!'

'To heal than to hurt!'

'Ohu!'

The man paused and looked at me. 'Will you honour our codes and, before all else, do no harm?'

The room watched me, silent, questioning.

'I will,' I answered, my voice thin in the charged space.

'Ohu-ohu-ohu!' they chanted.

'Bring forth the ram,' he commanded.

Two younger men came forward, holding an enormous ram skull on their shoulders. They stopped in front of me, the skull at eye level. They slowly turned it around to reveal a hole at the back. Someone handed the speaker an open can of beer, and he began to pour its contents into the skull. The crowd began to stir.

I wondered vaguely if they ever cleaned the skull.

The men put the skull to my lips.

'Ohu! Ohu! Ohu!'

The chanting resumed, softly at first, then rising to a crescendo as I gulped the cheap ale.

I managed to drink half the beer; the rest poured down the front of my overalls. The cheers grew to a roar.

A merry girl rushed forward and rubbed her fingers across my cheeks, leaving streaks of red. I was relieved to smell paint. Then I was swept into the air, carried on heads and arms from the house and into the backyard. The stuffy heat and manic chattering of the room was replaced with cool night air and the sound of music thumping from a large speaker perched on an outdoor table.

Finally, recognition! This was more like it!

But as the mob approached a muddy patch in the backyard, my euphoria evaporated.

'Where are you taking me?' I shouted helplessly, my voice drowned in the noise.

Then I was soaring through the air and splashing down into cold mud. Bodies started to splash around me, an odd medley of grunts and laughter. Soon other first-years were raining down like discarded spuds. Last of all was Pepper, who landed on me, sinking me deeper into the mud. She bounced back up, clean as a Persian cat, and hopped away giggling.

As the night progressed, I witnessed a series of boat races that had nothing to do with boats, mud-caked students resembling Uruk-hai, and a grown man peeing himself on purpose.

A fierce wrestling contest began between the horribly outnumbered first-years and the older students. Amidst the chaos, I noticed a boy I hadn't seen before. He was short and squat and was struggling in the mud against a much larger student. His wide-set, dark eyes had the tell-tale squint of someone used to wearing glasses. As he clenched his jaw and bared his teeth, I noticed a distinctive gap between his two front teeth.

The big man tossed the smaller chap to the ground, sitting on him triumphantly while his classmates cheered. It didn't look as though the hulk was going to give up his human stool anytime soon, so I took a run-up and launched myself at him as he revelled in his victory. I hit him shoulder-first, tackling him off the boy. We slid together along the muddy ground, me on top. I climbed off and went back over to pull the boy up, watching out of the corner of my eye for a counter-attack.

'Thanks!' he beamed, getting to his feet. 'I'm Don.' His teeth and eyes glowed white as he squinted at me from behind his muddy mask. We clasped hands.

'Marcus,' I told him. 'I think we are in for one hell of a ride, Don.'

Seconds later I was bulldozed off my feet and back into the mud by one of the girls. Don watched us for a moment and guessed that I didn't need to be rescued.

'Okay,' he called down to me, 'nice to meet you. I'll save you a seat in class.'

I managed to give him a thumbs-up before being rolled back down into the sludge. Maybe I needed rescuing after all.

Outside the anatomy lab, everyone looked different under the hallway's fluorescent lights. Mud and overalls had been replaced by clean faces and brand-new white lab coats. The only person I didn't have trouble recognising, with his mousy brown hair and pale skin, was Don. His eyes had relaxed now that his glasses were once more sitting comfortably on his nose, and he looked considerably more at home than he had in the wrestling pit. He moved over and glanced at the half-eaten sandwich in my hand.

'Is that . . .' — his eyes widened — '. . . MacKenzie bread?'

'Uh, yeah,' I confessed.

'Dude, those loaves are like four bucks fifty! Why are you eating your lunch anyway? It's nine a.m.'

'I heard the lab is three hours long,' I explained. 'I don't want to have a rumbling stomach while we cut up dogs . . .'

Don nodded solemnly and pulled out a Marmite sandwich, the black tar-like goop oozing from plain white slices of bread. 'This loaf was ninety-nine cents,' he told me glumly, still eyeing my sandwich.

I pulled it closer to my chest. Mercifully, just then the door opened and a tall, smiling man in his sixties gestured for us to come in. Don and I stuffed the rest of our sandwiches into our mouths and filed into the large room with the other students.

Soft gasps came from some of them as they took in their surroundings. There were 25 small steel tables spread throughout the room. On each one was a stiff, dead dog. Some were large, some small; there were Jack Russells, Rottweilers, terriers, collies and many other breeds. They stared blank-eyed as I walked slowly through the room.

'Choose one!' the lecturer called from the front. 'Get into groups of four. Choose wisely: this will be your cadaver for the next year and a half.'

I walked up to a chocolate Labrador with grey hair around his muzzle. Who had his family been? They must have been kind to have donated him to the vet school, trusting we would be respectful with him. Earlier, one of the older students had told me not to choose a Labrador, warning me that I'd spend most of my time trying to dissect through fat, so I moved on.

Next, I stopped in front of a white greyhound. He was lean, muscled and took up the entire tabletop. My Auckland classmates came over to join me, nodding their approval. Pepper looked down at the dog sadly.

'Poor guy,' she said, patting him with a gloved hand. 'I wonder if he just ran too slow.'

'Maybe he was adopted after his racing days and lived a full and happy life?' I suggested.

Our muted conversation came to an abrupt end as a girl fled the lab, tears streaking her cheeks. By now the room was mostly silent, except for a few low, muttered comments.

'Open your dissection kits!' the lecturer instructed.

I could see Don unzipping his kit as he stood next to the Labrador. I'd been so distracted by the sandwich antics that I'd forgotten to pass on the tip. He spotted me and gave me a happy nod, his glasses now sitting behind a large pair of safety goggles.

'Feel for the spine of the scapula,' the lecturer said. 'It runs down the shoulder towards the joint. That's where you need to make the first incision.' His head bobbed as the students obeyed.

I ran my finger down the bony ridge of the greyhound's scapula, or 'shoulder blade,' as you would more commonly say for a human. The dog was cold to the touch. The cadavers had been in the chiller before being laid out on the tables for us. I looked up at Olive.

'Did you really do this on human bodies at med school?' I asked her.

She nodded. 'You get used to it. We called our guy Fred.'

'Fred,' I echoed. 'What should we name our boy?'

We paused, then, when nothing was forthcoming, I picked up my scalpel.

'Do you mind if I do the first incision?' I asked. They nodded. I made a long cut behind the shoulder, then peeled a large flap of skin forward towards the dog's head to reveal the bright-red muscles of the shoulder. They were shiny from the formalin that had been injected into the cadavers to preserve them.

Pepper pointed to the muscle in front of the bony ridge on the scapula. 'I think that's the supraspinatus.'

I glanced up as another pale-faced student sped out of the room, one hand cupped to his mouth.

'I think that guy is about to throw up,' I said. The door swung shut behind him. As soon as I spoke, I realised that I was feeling a little light-headed, too. The room smelled of chemicals and flesh.

Pepper cut away the tendon on the muscle and lifted it, and as she did so a pale piece of connective tissue flicked up and hit my goggles, sticking there.

'Ahh!' I shouted. 'Gross!'

'Hello.'

I jumped at the man's voice. A large head had appeared over my shoulder.

'You're going to get much worse things flicked at your face on the job, I assure you.'

It was the lecturer. He circled around to face me, smiling. His head, sporting frizzy white hair, jutted forward.

'So,' he went on, 'what did you decide to name him?'

How had he heard us? He had been on the other side of the room.

'Mr Hoons,' I declared.

He looked at the greyhound, and then up at the rest of my group. 'Mr . . . Hoons?' He raised a bushy eyebrow.

'We're still working on a name,' Olive said.

Mr Hoons and our mad professor taught us as much as they could about canine anatomy over the next 18 months. As did Dobby the sheep, Ernest the chicken, Hodor the horse, and finally Francisco the fish.

Those years we spent diligently scurrying between labs and lectures in histology, pathology, pharmacology, physiology, virology, microbiology, radiology, dentistry, animal handling, genetics, medicine and surgery wouldn't be enough. They couldn't be enough. Nothing could quite prepare us for our next trial.

It was time to go out into the field.

CHAPTER THREE

THE ISLAND

THE THICK, HUMID AIR HIT US as soon as we stepped from the plane. In the distance, beyond the airfield, rich green jungle cloaked spiking mountains. Smiling locals playing Island music greeted us inside the terminal. The hulking man leading the musical trio dwarfed his ukulele.

'We are geniuses!' I declared to Don as we hauled our heavy suitcases up from the carousel. 'Doing our clinical placement on a tropical island is the best idea we've ever had.'

I thought of the other students, probably cramped in some dingy clinic experiencing an advanced state of vitamin D deficiency. My bag was heavy, filled with donated drugs from some generous vet clinics in New Zealand. A good number of them were prescription-only substances.

'Hey, uh, Don? How does this work, with all the drugs?' I asked, wondering why I hadn't thought to ask earlier.

Don shrugged. His bag was just as loaded. We put our bags up on the customs desk. A large, muscular man eyed us up.

'Kia orana. Anything to declare?' he asked.

'Yes. I have a bag full of drugs,' I told him.

He looked back at me coolly. I felt a sharp kick strike my shin. It was Don.

'We are here as volunteers at the vet clinic!' Don added hurriedly.

'Open the bags,' the man ordered.

We unzipped our suitcases to reveal an assortment of drug boxes, bottles and jars of various shapes and sizes. A shiny metal canister of isoflurane, an anaesthetic gas, sat glinting at the top of Don's pile. There was barely room for our clothes. The man glanced over the bags' contents. We held our breath.

''Kay.' He dismissed us with an absent wave of his hand.

We hauled our suitcases off the tables and dragged them towards the airport exit.

'Whoa. I hope they have a farm vet on this island, cos the mules just arrived, eh, Donny?' I laughed.

'Shut up,' Don growled. 'We're not even out of the airport yet, you blundering gumbie.'

'I'm pretty sure this island is so small they knew who we were as soon as we landed. I heard the prison here doesn't even have walls. The villagers just tell the guards if one of the prisoners is off wandering around and they come out and send them back. Plus, they do craft in there, whittling and stuff like that. Doesn't sound too bad.'

'I bet you five mangoes,' Don challenged, 'that's a yarn.'

I shook Don's hand confidently.

On a lawn scattered with coconuts in front of a simple, single-storey clinic waited the team we'd be assisting: the head vet, Lyn, a new graduate vet called Kari, and a handful of volunteers. One of them stood out from the rest. She was tall with olive skin, and smiled at me warmly before giving me a tight embrace. Mary-Anne was from California, and was putting in some volunteer hours before starting vet school there. I tried not to blush. Don shook his head at me, stifling a smile at my awkwardness.

'Welcome to our paradise!' Lyn announced abruptly. 'My first exam question for you is . . .' She paused dramatically. 'What is Long Island iced tea?'

Don and I looked at each other dumbly, then back at Lyn.

'Um, a drink?' Don tried.

'Not just a drink!' she declared. 'It's the best damn cocktail in the universe. And they make a blimmin' good one on this island. We're going to get one immediately! Mary-Anne, close the clinic at once.'

A week after those first introductions, I opened my eyes to see a large shar pei sitting beside my bed, his nose inches away from mine. A long globule of saliva hung glistening from his jowls, and his hot, fishy breath blasted my senses. Mary-Anne's face popped out from behind him, smiling.

'Good morning! It's ten a.m. How are you even still asleep?' she chastised. 'The cleaner was vacuuming right next to you, and there's like ten dogs in there.' She gestured towards the kennels, where a band of dogs barked a deafening medley.

A snippet from the night before flashed through my mind. I was leaning out the back of an open-sided bus with a thatched roof, trying to high-five someone on a motorbike. The lead vet had a strict 'no Long Island iced tea, no surgery for you the next day' policy. For the third time that week, I had obliged. The only issue was I didn't share her veteran British liver.

I felt a small surge of panic. 'Wait — am I meant to be in surgery?' I asked, my eyes widening, head throbbing.

Mary-Anne grinned at me. 'Nah, it's your day off! I just thought you might be dying. I gotta go back.' She trotted off, the shar pei in tow.

I dawdled to the kitchen in search of water. I was halfway through a bottle when Don burst in. 'Where's Lyn?' he demanded, glancing around the house.

'I dunno,' I gurgled. 'What's up?'

'Kari's in surgery and she can't find the cat's uterus.'

'I can help,' I said.

Don raised his eyebrows. We were in our third year of university and had barely done a single surgery.

'What are you going to do, dive in there with your snorkel?'

I headed towards the surgery room. As I opened the heavy door and stepped into the cool air of the only air-conditioned room in the clinic Kari looked up; she had a finger in the cat's abdomen, searching for the uterus, which was to be removed. She was flustered and clearly disappointed that I wasn't Lyn, the head vet. I stepped up to the table and lifted a corner of the surgery drape.

'I checked that,' a nurse snapped, irritated.

I parted the fur just below the cat's bottom, and two small fluffy balls looked back at me.

'It's a boy,' I said, dropping the drape and leaving the surgery room. I didn't know how to do surgery yet, but I had spent a few days with Mary-Anne, sexing the kittens. She would hold them up and quiz me. I was hilariously bad at the seemingly simple task at first, but soon got a grip on it. It was mostly an excuse just to hang around with her, but today my feline studies had paid off.

The day before, though, things had not gone so well. A man had brought a wild cat to the clinic, and as I was the only one there at the time, I'd decided I could take care of things. We were running a desexing programme to reduce the populations of wild cats and dogs on the island, and the man had spent a lot of time and effort catching the cat and bringing it into the clinic. He sat the cage down on the dirt in front of the outdoor kennels. I knelt and peered in. Two wild green eyes stared back at me. I rose and picked up a towel from the shelf.

'Are you sure you can do this?' the man asked, doubt clear in his eyes.

'Yeah, mate. No worries, I got this,' I assured him.

I mean, after all, how hard could it be to pin down a wild

cat and throw it into one of our cages? It's a tiny, 3-kilogram little critter after all . . . I tipped the cage on its back, so that the door was facing the sky, then I opened it, tentatively peering in. The hunched feline glared up at me, hissing and spitting from the bottom of the cage. I dropped the towel on it. The cat fell silent.

I went to reach in, then hesitated. 'More towels, please,' I said with the air of a surgeon asking for his scalpel.

The man passed me two more towels, and I dropped them onto the cat. I stared down at the pile of towels in the cage, an enraged wild cat somewhere in the mix. The man looked nervous.

Man, this guy needed to chill. I slowly put my hands down into the cage. A low droning began to reverberate from the centre of the towel ball as I wrapped my hands around it, gripping tightly. As I slowly extracted my prize, the ball of tooth and muscle went rigid in my grip, like a loaded spring ready to fire.

'Open that cage. Please!' This time I sounded less like a surgeon and more like a frightened boy. I gestured to a kennel cage. The towel bomb exploded in my hands. A black head burst from the top, teeth bared, ears flat. The cat screeched and hissed.

I held the towels as tightly as I could. The determined beast pushed down with its feet and freed half of its body. I couldn't pull the towel back over the cat without releasing what little grasp I had left. The man stared, his eyes wide, and took a step back. I looked at him wildly, pleading for him to do something.

He began fumbling with the cage latch. The cat twisted in my grip, sensing freedom was close. I had seconds to act. I ran towards the open clinic door, the writhing cat held out in front of me. With one last thrash, the cat flew from the towels and landed on the ground in a crouch. Then, in a flash, it was gone — a black streak vanishing into the thick jungle.

I stared into the bush for a moment. Please, come back? I looked from the empty towels in my hands, now covered in black fur, to the man. He didn't meet my eyes. There was nothing much to say.

'Uh, sorry . . . sir,' I tried.

Without a word, he picked up his cage and left.

Now, on my day off, I winced at the still-painful memory as I walked over to the puppy pen. Those little fuzz-balls always cheered me up as they tumbled and rolled about, chewing on each other fondly. I grabbed an armful of them, bundled them against my chest and made my way across the road to the beach.

'Swimming lesson time, kids!' I told them.

The white sand was warm beneath my feet as I passed under the palm trees and towards the clear turquoise water. I put the pups down into the shallows and watched them bound around happily. Then I scooped one back up and waded further out into the warm water, out to where she couldn't touch the bottom. She clung onto me tightly. I let her go in the water and she swam to me. She scrambled up my chest, her claws scratching at me. 'Ow, lady!' I scolded. Red claw-marks now criss-crossed my chest.

'Hey, mister.' Mary-Anne stood on the beach in a sky-blue scrub top. I felt a tightness high in my chest. 'I need a hand to feed Luey. But you look like you have your hands full there, huh?' she added with a wry smile. 'I hope those claw-marks are from the puppy. I heard about your antics yesterday . . .'

Blast. What *had* I done last night?

'You know, there's another cat out there breeding in that jungle, thanks to you!' She laughed.

I chuckled, embarrassed.

'No, no, it's fine. I was just about finished here anyway . . .' I gathered up the puppies. 'Let's go.'

Mary-Anne led me back across the road. We returned the puppies to their little wrestling arena and made our way over to Luey the spaniel's hospital pen. He was lying on his side, his eyes flicking from side to side. He tried to lift his head when he heard us, but he couldn't, and it flopped back down onto the blanket.

'What's wrong with him?' I asked her.

'You tell me, you're the vet,' she replied, a glint in her eye.

'I have about fifty more exams to pass before I can say that,' I pointed out.

I opened the pen door and knelt down next to Luey to examine him. His body was floppy. Flaccid paralysis. His pupils continued to flick rapidly from side to side. Nystagmus. Maybe his vestibular system — which involves the inner ear and helps with balance — was affected?

'Could it be botulism?' I ventured. I knew animals could ingest bacteria that produced the botulinum toxin, usually from rotting animals or bones. That could make them go all floppy, like this guy was.

'It's fish poisoning,' she told me.

'I've never heard of that. Which fish?'

'It's not about the fish — it's a toxic alga that grows in the fish. If animals ingest it, they get like this.' She pointed at Luey.

I looked at him again. 'Poor thing . . . Can he survive?'

'If we take good care of him. His body needs time to clear the toxin.'

With that, she joined me in the pen. She mixed some dog food with water to make a paste. I elevated Luey's body on some blankets so his head hung down, to stop fluid from running down into his lungs. As I cradled his head, Mary-Anne slowly syringed the food onto his tongue. He was still able to move it and swallow a little.

'Good boy,' she soothed. 'Part of our work is to educate people on the island.' She slowly syringed another mouthful into Luey. 'We need to tell them that feeding raw fish to the dogs can be fatal.'

'You should educate new arrivals here about Lyn's Long Island iced teas, too. The symptoms are strikingly similar.'

Mary-Anne let out a warm burst of laughter. 'Well, at least you know how this poor guy feels.'

The next day we returned to Luey's pen. This time we took him out and tried to walk him. His legs were still limp, and they couldn't bear any weight, so we wrapped a towel under his belly and lifted him, Mary-Anne standing on one side, and me on the other. We walked him a few steps along the grass this way, his legs wobbling. He was desperate to walk, but his feet weren't responding. After a few lengths of the small lawn, we gave him a rest.

Luey's progress was slow, but day by day he began to bear more weight as he walked. With the help of the rest of the team at the clinic, we repeated his feeding and exercise routines for five days until he finally took a few unsteady steps on his own. It was a few more days before he could eat and walk normally again.

Once Lyn was satisfied with his condition, a local couple arrived to pick him up. They were overjoyed to see Luey recovered. The woman handed Don a large box filled with mangoes and bananas. Still on a student budget, Don and I had been living off these tokens of gratitude for the past few weeks, along with canned fish. The clean food and sun had left us glowing with health. Don's hair was shinier, although I guessed his liver resembled a chewed boot.

'Chur-chur!' Lyn appeared, holding up a bottle of gin. Mary-Anne was standing beside her, an apologetic look on her face. 'This is a time for celebration!'

Don and I groaned in unison.

I was going to need the same gentle treatment as Luey if I stayed on this island much longer.

Mary-Anne and I walked on the beach beneath a startling canvas of stars.

Mary-Anne spoke first. 'We're not going to see each other again, are we?' The question hung in the air. I was going back home to finish my degree, and she would be starting her own studies in California. It had been only a month, but spending every day together had brought us close.

'I'll miss you, Mary-Anne,' I offered.

'Marcus!' Don shouted from the street. He paused when he saw us holding hands. 'The taxi is here . . .' he finished lamely. 'Sorry,' he added, and turned and walked back up to the road.

We followed Don to where the taxi waited. I wanted to kiss her, but would doing so mean I would just miss her even more? We were approaching the rest of the group, and my window was closing. I stopped and turned to face her.

'Maybe we'll cross paths some day?' The emptiness of the words resounded with a dull clang.

Mary-Anne smiled sadly and pulled me into a tight embrace. Don called out that we would miss the plane if we didn't get a move-on. Maybe I wanted to miss the plane. Maybe I could just stay here forever with Mary-Anne, eating mangoes and drinking Long Island iced tea.

I pictured the pile of textbooks waiting for me on my desk at home. As much as I wanted to stay and live off mangoes, I couldn't. As much as I longed to abandon those books, they needed to be read. It was time to go. Back to university. Back to reality.

CHAPTER FOUR

HAT THIEF

DAIRY CATTLE GRAZED on the low hills, their black-and-white bodies contrasting with the rich green grass. We had been back in New Zealand only a few days and Don and I were driving to a clinic in the North Island. It was the beginning of spring placements. The idea was for us to assist as many cows with calving as we could before going out into the 'real' world as qualified vets. I wasn't so sure I wanted to go out into the real world. I liked my current world.

Don parked, and we walked in through the staff entrance at the back. One of our classmates and a young man I didn't recognise greeted us.

'Hello. I'm Tom,' he said warmly. 'I study in Ireland and I'm here on placement, too. Guess what?' He held up a pair of knitted hats, which matched the ones he and our classmate were already wearing and sported the logo of the clinic we were placed at. 'Free hats!' He handed me and Don a hat each, and we popped them onto our heads.

'Nice to meet you,' I said, 'and thanks for the hat. Excuse

me for a second.' I needed the bathroom. I walked into the hallway, where I spotted two older men coming from the opposite direction. One was large with short grey hair, the other couldn't have been an inch over five feet and had a shiny bald head. It was the clinic manager and the head vet, Jan. As we converged, their smiles shifted to frowns. They stopped in front of me, looking me over.

'What makes you think you have the right?' the taller man snapped, his face flushing to a dangerous hue.

'The . . . right?' I stammered, perplexed.

'Yes. The *right*,' he bit off the word. 'You are a guest in our clinic — those hats are for clients.' He spoke as though I was hard of hearing. 'Are you a client?'

I looked back at the pair dumbly. 'Not . . . that I am aware of . . . no.' I felt ill. What a terrible start.

'Not that you're *aware* of?' His voice grew louder. 'Of course you're not a damn client, you're a student!'

Jan hadn't spoken a word, but was also frowning at me. I heard footsteps behind me. Thank God: one of the others was coming to explain the misunderstanding. I turned to see Don approaching, a solemn expression on his face. He was no longer wearing his hat. He walked past me and stood alongside the angry pair, frowning along with them. He shook his head at me, his lips pressed together in a disapproving line.

I stared, disbelieving of Don's betrayal.

I turned back to the men. 'I was given the impression we were allowed to wear them. This is just a mistake . . . look, everyone thought the same thing,' I finished lamely.

I led the brooding men back into the room. Maybe if they saw that the other students were also confused about it . . .?

But the other two had clearly overheard the scolding and thrown their hats back in the box. They looked up at us from their freshly opened textbooks with wide, innocent eyes.

'Enough!' the clinic manager boomed, clearly fed up. 'Don't let me catch you stealing again.' The two men turned on their heels and left.

'You lot are unbelievable!' I said.

'Hey,' Don raised his palms defensively, 'it's not our fault you're some kind of kleptomaniac, Marcus.' I would have lunged for him, but someone was coming back down the hall.

'You. Hat thief.' Jan pointed a stubby finger at me. 'You're with me this morning.'

Three cows were standing in a holding pen outside. Two of them had their heads up and were watching us, and the other, rough-coated and skinny, had her head down. We had sat in uncomfortable silence on the drive to the farm, so it was a relief to now finally meet the patients.

'Let's get them through to the crush and see what's going on,' Jan said.

A crush allows vets to safely examine an animal without it moving around, and this crush was a narrow railed lane with a metal bar at the end. The bar could be pulled across to hold the cow's head in place once she'd poked her neck past it.

I walked into the pen behind Jan and we approached the cows, whistling and waving to move them along. Jan's head was about level with the cows' backsides; how he managed to handle the big Friesian cattle was beyond me.

We got the sick cow into the crush, and Jan handed me a thermometer. I walked up behind her and lifted her tail to take her rectal temperature. It was high. Her hip bones stood out sharply on either side of her tail base. Jan handed me a long plastic glove. The farmer had arrived by now, and was leaning on a rail watching me.

'When did she calve?' I asked him. Knowing how long since she had given birth would help give me an idea of what was going on.

The farmer straightened, his wispy hair catching the breeze. He pulled a grubby notebook out from the chest pocket in his overalls and fingered through it. 'About two weeks ago.'

I pulled the plastic glove up over my arm and put my hand into the cow's birth canal. I wanted to check for signs of damage from the calving, and for any smelly discharge that would indicate an infection. When I removed my hand, it was covered in a mucky brown liquid. It stank. She had an infected uterus. I held up my dripping hand to Jan.

'So, what will you do now?' he asked me.

'Well, she has clinical metritis, so . . .' I paused, considering the options. 'Antibiotics to clear the infection, and an anti-inflammatory to help with pain and get her fever down.'

'Good. But does she have mastitis? A heart problem?'

'I don't know.'

'No, of course not. Because you haven't finished examining the cow,' he said. 'Just because she has metritis doesn't mean she hasn't got something else wrong with her.'

I checked her udder, putting my hand on the back quarters, then the front. It wasn't swollen, and when I squeezed the teats pure white milk came from them. Her gut sounds, breathing and heart were okay.

I looked at her eyes, they were a little sunken.

'I think she might be dehydrated, too,' I added, tentatively.

'So, what should we do about that?' Jan asked, showing surprising patience considering I had robbed him just that morning.

'We could give her oral fluids?' I suggested.

Jan nodded. Maybe I was making up for earlier? But judging by the look on Jan's face, I still had a long way to go.

I went and got a bucket of lukewarm water and mixed in a pack of electrolytes from Jan's truck. I threw a steel pump in the bucket and picked up a long rubber tube. As I took it out, I noticed a pair of stilts sitting behind it. I pictured Jan walking around on the stilts, juggling fire in front of a crowd at the circus. His part-time job?

By the time I returned to the crush, Jan had already drawn up the injections. He eyed me as I carried the equipment up to the cow's head.

'Do you know how to use that?' he asked.

'I did it once at university . . .'

Jan came over and stood next to the cow's head, facing the same way she was. He reached his arm over her nose and hooked his hand into the side of her mouth, lifting her head up remarkably easily for a man of his size.

'Hold her head up with your right arm and feed the tube with your left. Got it?' He regarded me intently to make sure I understood.

I nodded. We swapped places. I reached over and put my hand in her mouth. She thrashed her head from side to side, throwing me around. I finally managed to pull her head up, which settled her a bit. I was panting heavily when Jan passed me the feeding tube. The farmer was openly amused by my flailing. The tube fed nicely, and we pumped her rumen, the cow's first stomach, with two buckets of the electrolyte mix. Jan looked pleased. Next, I gave her the penicillin and an anti-inflammatory, injecting them into her thick neck muscle, one on each side.

'Do you think she'll survive?' I asked.

'You can never know for sure,' he told me. 'All you can do is give them the best chance possible, the rest is up to them, and, well,' he winked at the farmer, 'the farmer giving the follow-up—'

He was cut short by a clang from the pen where the two other cows had been waiting. One of the cows was escaping. She'd pushed open the gate and had seized her opportunity, trotting down the lane towards the road, her udder swinging happily as she ran. Jan swore.

'You didn't close the bloody gate!' he shouted back at me, as he dashed after the cow. He continued to curse as he ran down the lane, his little legs scurrying under him. The cow sped up. Without stopping, she turned onto the main road and continued her dash. Jan continued his chase. The profanities flying from his mouth grew fainter as his shining bald head receded into the distance.

While I stood there doing nothing, the farmer mounted his motorbike. He sped off and rounded the cow up, bringing her back up the road, along the track, and then to her pen. Jan walked behind, puffing. He didn't look at me.

When we climbed back into the truck, the morning's uncomfortable silence had returned.

As we drove, I tried desperately to think of a way to start up a conversation, to get things back on a more even keel.

Finally, I blurted out, 'Are you in the circus?'

Jan's head turned so red that the heat it was emitting began fogging the car window beside it.

If I failed this placement, I would have to go back for another two weeks — a scenario that was beginning to look increasingly likely at this point.

A few weeks later I sat in my room staring at an envelope. The sender's address was Jan's clinic. I stared at it, imagining my picture on their wall, darts protruding at various angles from my face. The rest of my farm visits there were with the other vets, presumably for the sake of Jan's sanity. One of them had explained that his stilts were for reaching cows' back ends inside the dairy shed. I took a deep breath and tore the envelope open.

Satisfactory.

'Yes!' I shouted triumphantly.

'What?' Don popped his head into my room.

'I passed,' I announced.

'Was that the clinic where you stole the hats and made that little bald vet run after a cow?' He spouted the sentence like the whole thing was one word.

'I didn't steal anything!'

Don ducked as one of my shoes flew at him.

'Hey, man, chill. Save your energy,' he said. 'You're going to be dancing in front of six hundred hungry women tonight, remember?'

How could I forget? I looked over at the gold Spartan helmet sitting proudly on my desk, a mohawk of red hair sprouting from the top. I had spent weeks sculpting papier mâché to get it right.

'The footsteps of the bold echo into eternity, my friend,' I said solemnly.

Don shook his head, chuckling. 'You're in for it, buddy. You thought the wounds from that tomcat the other day were bad.'

The event he was talking about was, of course, Mr Vet — the vet school's infamous male beauty pageant.

'You think you'll fare any better?' I teased.

He scowled. 'I'm only competing because of you, traitor.'

'That's what you get for that saga with the hat.'

Don stomped off.

We were nearing the end of vet school. The willing men

from our class had already stepped up in previous years, flaunting themselves in front of the lusty crowd. This year my name had been drawn in the ballot. My time had come.

There was no way out of this one.

CHAPTER FIVE

MR VET

FOUR WEEKS EARLIER, before the dreaded Mr Vet event, a walrus-moustached professor had been rambling about antibiotics when the vet school student president burst into the lecture hall.

'We need two champions to represent your class for Mr Vet this year!' he'd announced. There were only a handful of men in the class, sitting huddled together like endangered penguins. The ones who had already done their duty leaned back comfortably, eyeing the uninitiated with glee. Don and I put our heads down, trying to become invisible. I could feel the increasing number of eyes on me and my anxiety rising. A murmuring slowly transitioned into a low chant. 'Mar-cus, Mar-cus, Mar-cus . . .'

I kept my head down. Dancing around in my underwear in front of half the university was not on my agenda this month.

'Mar-cus, Mar-cus, Mar-cus!' the chanting grew to a roar.

I glanced up at the president, who turned his hands up, apologetically. The pressure was unbearable. I had to do something, put my foot down and end this madness. I burst to my feet. The chanting stopped, and 100 sets of eyes stared at me expectantly.

'I'll do it!' I turned and pointed, my finger trembling. 'IF DON DOES IT WITH ME!'

The class went ballistic. Don's eyes widened in disbelief. I danced manically in momentary glory before the lecturer bustled the president out and called for order. Don's head had sunk down onto his desk. I'd just signed us up for the most humiliating event in university history.

'I hate you,' Don muttered, his cheek squished against his workbook.

The air was electric in the changing room. When Don came stumbling back in, he was panting, his cheeks flushed. He was covered in silver glitter, only a leopard-print G-string between himself and the world.

'A word of advice,' he gasped. 'Don't go down off the stage — they will try to pull your undies off.'

Pepper, who was part of my supporting cast, had just finished wrapping herself in a black sheet and was spinning a sword artfully. She saw the look of horror on my face and picked up a flask, extending it to me. 'Are you sure you don't want a drink?'

I pushed her hand away.

She put a supportive hand on my knee. 'You've got this, okay?'

'Are you wearing the chest pad?' I asked. My voice sounded pinched and nervous.

Pepper feigned offence. 'What makes you think I need to pad my chest?'

Just then a woman from the class below me stuck her head through the door. 'You ready?' she asked, looking me up and down. 'Wow, nice . . . armour.'

She was assigned to escort me onto the stage. Don and the other contestants had had an escort, too, half for show and half to keep the wobblier competitors on their feet.

The golden helmet was on my head, the blood-red plume standing proud. Matching plated greaves were on my legs and I was clad in a brown loincloth and a full-length red silk cape. I was brandishing a 7-foot spear, and a sword hung sheathed on my belt. Strapped to my arm was a shield made from a rubbish bin lid spray-painted gold. My chest and thighs were bare. I felt like a Spartan. I was ready for war. Around the room stood my friends, 15 'Persian soldiers'.

'You all look great,' I said. 'See you on the field of battle!' They cheered as my escort, wearing a sparkling gold dress, entered the room, took my arm, and led me to the stage.

'And now,' she announced, 'we have Marcus Taylor, who says . . . "I will stand and die with King Leonidas!" Whatever the hell that means! Let's just hope he does something better than Simon's Rowan Atkinson impersonation last year.'

The audience laughed like a pack of hyenas, then hushed. She grabbed my arm. I was shaking.

'Play the music,' I instructed the sound desk, trying to swallow the lump in my throat. 'O Fortuna' boomed from the speakers. I braced.

STAAAAAATUUUU VAAAAAARIABIIILIS.
Semper crescis . . .

I walked further out onto the stage, feeling the heat as the bright lights struck my skin. Hundreds of faces filled my vision as I looked out at the packed auditorium and was met with whoops and cheers. I raised my shield and spear and shook them at the crowd, raising a few more cheers. My flatmates hooted at me from the front row. I twirled my spear as the first wave of Persians crept onto the stage, knives in their mouths.

'Behind you!' someone obligingly called from the masses.

I spun around and ran at my foes, disembowelling the first with a straight thrust into his stomach. He rolled onto the stage clutching his gut, groaning dramatically. I danced back from a knife slash, and then jabbed my spear through the attacker's throat — or at least past the side of their neck as they stood side-on to the crowd. The crowd was well into their boxes of beers and easy to entertain. I hit the third attacker across the head with the back of my spear. Standing over them, I drove my spear between chest and arm.

This felt good. As wave after wave of Persian warriors ran onto the stage, I ran them through with my spear. Finally, someone got hold of my weapon and snatched it from my hands. I drew my sword and slashed their throat, roaring savagely. The crowd whooped.

'Show no mercy!' someone called drunkenly.

Then Big Darryl climbed onto the stage. He was six foot four and wielding a huge axe. A real axe. This was one move we couldn't mess up. I tried not to think of Darryl swigging rum from his flask in the dressing room earlier.

He swung the axe in great wild arcs. There was a manic look in his eyes. Did he genuinely want to murder me? Before I could decide, he drew the axe back as if he was going to chop down a tree. Surging forward, he swung at me, the axe whirling in a deadly arc. I leaned back in the deepest limbo I could summon. The axe brushed the tip of my nose. A woosh of air hit my face. I righted myself, and, before he could take another swing, I stabbed him in the groin, hard. He winced and fell.

'Bastard,' he muttered, dropping to the floor.

The only one left was Pepper, who was holding her sword out in front of her. We sparred, blocking and slashing until I had backed her all the way down to the end of the catwalk. I knocked her sword aside and she shuffled back, her heels hanging over the edge.

The music stopped.

'Please!' Pepper pleaded. 'This . . . this is madness!'

'Madness? This is SPARTA!' I kicked her straight in her padded chest. She flew off the stage, crashing into a mat below. I looked up at the crowd and raised my sword. There was a short pause, and then—

A deafening roar. They screamed and clapped. My

adrenaline surged as I stood on the stage, which was now littered with the bodies of felled warriors.

The shouting went on and on. I bowed, and then pulled Pepper back up onto the stage. My friends clambered to their feet and took bows of their own. We buzzed from the stage, ecstatic.

After Simon's disaster last year, I'd been imagining the worst. I made a quick costume change and returned to the stage with my guitar. Dressed in a toga, I performed a song by Shaggy and soon the entire auditorium was singing along.

A short time later, I was lined up with the other Mr Vet competitors. Their performances had been impressive. One had eaten a raw ram's testicle. Don had done a magic show, clad scandalously. Ribbon dancing had featured, and there had even been a jazz flute solo. I was really up against it.

'Without further ado . . . it is time to name our champion!' The audience screamed, until the emcee finally subdued them into silence.

He held the mic close to his mouth. 'And for the first time ever . . . we have a tie, naming not one, but two champions . . . Congratulations — Marcus and Don!'

The crowd screamed once more as the yellow Mr Vet sash was draped over us both. The other competitors wobbled from the stage, leaving Don and me raising our arms to the crowd.

‘You see, Donny,’ I shouted in his ear as we waved, ‘it was all for the greater good!’

All those weeks of papier mâché and fight training had actually paid off. Not to mention spending all my grocery money on a silk cape. He jabbed me with an elbow.

‘I am still going to murder you!’

‘I’ll buy you a beer!’ We leapt off the stage, the sash binding us together, the bandage for my betrayal.

CHAPTER SIX

OUTBACK

MY EXPERIENCE IN THE COOK ISLANDS had been so great that I booked another clinic placement overseas as soon as I could. Reading an exciting book about a young man who'd got lost in the Australian desert had got my heart set on exploring the vast land of orange sunsets, horses and wild cattle. So I found a vet clinic deep in the Australian wilderness. I was going to the Outback.

Unfortunately, right before I was due to depart I caught a nasty stomach bug from some sick calves. I could barely move, eat or drink, but somehow I managed to stagger onto the plane and was on my way.

Once we'd crossed the Australian coastline, we flew over flat brown land for what seemed an eternity. I stared vacantly out the window, my eyes following the path of a silvery river snaking its way beneath the plane, its twists and turns mirroring my stomach's internal gurglings. Finally, we landed on a lonely runway, shimmering in the heat.

After a long taxi ride, I reclaimed my heavy hiking bag from the boot and swung it up onto my back. I stumbled towards a distant sports field of bone-dry grass surrounded by gum trees, whose sun-baked leaves clattered in the wind. Horses were running around the pitch, their riders holding short sticks.

What on earth were they doing? I was so dehydrated and unwell that I could not completely dismiss the possibility that I was hallucinating.

A white-bearded Aboriginal man who was sitting on a low fence beside the parking lot started shouting at me.

'Ayyha! Ayy! Maite! You goin' wokabout, mate? Yurona wokabout, eh? Ha!' he hollered, his voice as rough as rusted iron.

I pondered his question, and for a moment the only sounds were my boots crunching the dry leaves underfoot and the riders' shouts in the distance.

'In fact, yes indeed. I am!' I answered cheerfully as I passed.

He cheered and raised his can of beer to me. Excellent.

A few moments later I'd made it over to where the vet and his family were waiting for me.

Closer inspection revealed that the sticks I'd seen the riders gripping resembled lacrosse sticks, and they — vet and family included — were well immersed in a game.

One man threw a ball to another using the cradle at the end of his stick, then the catcher galloped towards a mounted goalkeeper positioned in front of what looked like a hockey goal. There was a semicircle around the goal that the riders couldn't enter. Inside the goal area, the keeper manoeuvred his horse backwards and forwards with just his knees in order to block the goal. The attacker flung the ball like a bullet past the keeper and scored, wheeling his horse around triumphantly in an arc of dust.

In the ensuing pause in play while the players regrouped, the vet spotted me standing there with my backpack and turned his horse towards me. Three men in their early twenties trotted up behind him. They stopped their horses next to his, the animals tossing their heads impatiently.

I was feeling sick, tired and overheated. The men and horses were covered in sweat and dust, but the men eyed me coolly from beneath the brims of their hats. I was trying not to keel over in the breeze as the sun scorched my bare head from above and the hot ground cooked me from below.

The vet slid from his horse, landing in the dust with a soft thud. He was short and stocky, with leathery, wrinkled skin. His arms were knotted with the muscles of a man who never stopped working.

'You need a hat,' he told me flatly, gripping my hand in an iron handshake. 'John Kay.' His hand felt like a rhino's hide. He pointed to each of the men, introducing them as his sons. They gave curt nods, and I nodded back.

'What sport is that?' I asked, pointing towards the field.

The boys looked at each other, bemused. John's expression remained deadpan.

'It's polocrosse, mate. Big deal here.' John had the strongest Aussie twang I had ever heard. 'We'll get you riding before long.'

An hour later the horses were loaded into the back of the truck, and we were driving towards the town. The road headed off in a straight line over the horizon. The road trains — huge trucks, with five or six trailers in tow — coming in the other direction shook our horse truck as they sped past. Scattered across the ground were termite mounds, each twice the height of a man, standing like miniature mountains between the dry scrub and spindly trees.

I snapped to attention as we suddenly drove into thick smoke. Tall flames leapt and danced in the bush around us, smoke billowing from the trees.

'Jeez! Fire!' I warned them.

The boys sniggered. 'That's a burn-off, mate. No problem,' the oldest one said.

A moment later we were past the fire, and the smoke cleared. I stayed quiet for the rest of the drive. I still hadn't eaten, and I no longer trusted myself to speak.

We arrived in the small town late at night. As the horse truck pulled into John's property, bugs zipped in front of the headlights and bullfrogs croaked from the darkness. The horses stamped and whinnied, eager to be out of the truck.

The youngest son walked two horses down the ramp and handed me their lead ropes. The brothers then gathered the other horses, and we walked them towards the stables. It felt good to have a rope in each hand and horses walking calmly on either side of me; maybe this wasn't going to be so har—

Something was tugging at my feet.

I stumbled forward in rapid tiny steps as some strange force held my feet together. I desperately tried to stay upright, but it was hopeless — I hit the ground face-first with a thud. The horses and boys alike stopped and stared at me, perplexed.

I clambered back to my feet, covered in dust. I looked down at my feet; in my haste I had managed to lace my boots together. My horses stopped, their lead ropes hanging freely, and waited patiently for me to compose myself. I could hear the boys trying to suppress their laughter as I corrected the lace disaster and regained control of the horses.

An orange sun sat low on the horizon as John handed me a lead rope. I looked around, confused. There wasn't a horse in sight.

'You're going to learn to ride,' John announced. 'People who live around here and can't ride are useless.' He watched me. 'You don't want to be useless, do you?'

'Certainly not.'

'Okay. Go catch a horse,' he directed. 'There are forty of them in that forest; I'm sure you can find at least one.'

I looked out at the apparently empty forest.

'I'm not cruel — here.' He handed me a black bucket, half full of grain. 'Off ya go.' With that, he was gone.

I dawdled into the trees with a sinking heart. This was starting to feel a lot like the book that had prompted me to take this placement in the first place: a boy had got separated from the other cattle workers and had wandered the Outback for weeks, hopelessly lost and surviving by eating grass. It wasn't uncommon for people to get lost in the Outback. Circling endlessly, disoriented in the monotonous terrain, it didn't take long before they died of thirst.

I looked down into my bucket. Sure, I could survive on dry horse-feed, but what would I drink?

After I'd been walking for five minutes, I was already considering drinking my own pee. I also hadn't seen any horses. Was this some kind of initiation?

My feet snapped dead sticks as I trudged across the cracked ground. If I kept the sun on my left, I would at least be able to walk the same direction back. Plus, if there were horses here there must be fences. Then again, these properties were huge, thousands of square kilometres, so maybe they didn't need fences.

A wallaby shot past me, bouncing through the scrub. Overhead, dozens of enormous black vultures cruised on the thermals, their silhouettes stark against the blue sky.

Bringing my eyes back down to the trees, I saw movement. A dozen horses were making their way through the trees, eyeing my bucket. They surrounded me, shouldering each other out of the way to get to the horse feed. Their breath was hot on my face and arms as they huffed and stomped impatiently. The grain was rapidly vanishing; I needed to catch one before I had nothing to hold their interest.

As a grey stallion dipped his nose into the bucket, I threw a rope over his neck, reaching across his front to retrieve the other end. 'Gotcha.'

He looked at me, annoyed, but otherwise yielding. I put his halter on and walked him back the way I'd come.

I emerged from the trees to find John working in his shed. He looked up, clearly surprised to see me arriving back with my prize.

'I didn't think you'd get one,' he said, handing me a saddle.

I looked at it blankly.

John frowned impatiently. 'Like this.' He threw the saddle over the stallion's back and fixed and adjusted the straps, his fingers deft. 'His name's Tucker. Hop on.' I put a foot in the near stirrup and stepped up, swinging my back leg over. 'Good. Off you go.' He marched off again before I could tell him I didn't know how to ride.

Tucker flicked his ears at a fly. I looked out at the vast expanse of dry dirt and scrappy trees. At least there weren't too many things to crash into. The sun was a deep orange, now setting behind the flatlands that stretched around me as far as the eye could see. It was quiet, peaceful.

I gently tapped my heels against Tucker's stomach. He didn't move.

'Yarrr!' I tried. Nothing. I kicked harder and he immediately walked forward.

We plodded along at a casual pace.

'All right, Tucker. This isn't so bad. Good boy!'

He started to trot. I began to bounce in the saddle, so I sat up and tried to time my downward bounce with every second bump of his gait. It was like music. I just needed to count and stay in time with him. We trotted into a clearing and down the middle of an old airstrip. Tucker, sensing the extra space, began to speed up a little. A group of wallabies bounded past.

'Chaaaahuuuuu!' I shouted triumphantly. Tucker started to speed up even more. 'Whoa. WHOA, Tucker! Tucker!'

Tucker moved into a canter, the new gait throwing me off balance. His big strides threw me around in the saddle until I fell forward onto his neck like a limp doll. My boots were slipping from the stirrups, and, before I could adjust, one foot fell free. I gripped a handful of Tucker's mane. The hard ground raced beneath me.

'No! Tucker!' I finally managed to sit up again, and leaned back, pulling on the reins desperately.

Tucker slowed to a trot and then a walk, and I panted from the adrenaline dump.

'Listen, Tucker. I know you want to race those wallabies, but I don't know how to ride a horse, so you'll have to blimmin' wait,' I told him.

Tucker snorted and continued to sedately plod down the runway.

Over the course of the following month, Tucker taught me to ride. I would even learn to pick up and throw a polocrosse ball while on horseback before I left Australia.

I didn't know it at the time, but those weeks riding and

handling horses would be priceless, teaching me how to behave around them and remain calm. Horses and their owners can sense nerves a mile away, and neither of them wants a nervous vet.

The next day I visited the nearby small Outback township for the first time. I had almost reached Mr Kay's vet clinic when I saw a phone booth with a large woman inside it, screaming. As I got closer the volume increased, and I could begin to make out a colourful stream of profanities. After every second word, the Aboriginal woman took the phone receiver from her ear and smashed it against the machine.

She must have sensed me staring at her, because she spun around and roared at me, 'RAAAaaaaahhh! Mother FU—'

I hurried on.

Alongside a nearby river there were tents huddled among the bushes, beer cans scattered around them like fallen soldiers. Two thin Aboriginal men in ragged shorts and singlets yelled at me from across the street.

'Aye!' one of the men shouted. 'Aye, you!' He called again, louder, making sure he had my attention. 'Fuck you!' They laughed. Their eyes were wild; they were high. I sped up again, heading to the clinic.

I soon discovered that the unrest I'd witnessed was the daily norm. There was a vast divide between the white locals and the Aboriginals in the community, and, sadly, overt racism was just fuel on the fire.

One of the nurses gave me a flying tour of the set-up when I arrived at the clinic and I spent the rest of the morning seeing consults with the companion-animal vet.

When I eventually bumped into John he told me I needed to be at his runway at 5 a.m. sharp the next morning. I knew the spot well; it was where I'd almost tumbled from Tucker's back. We were going to be heading even deeper into the vast expanse of the Australian Outback.

CHAPTER SEVEN

FURTHER OUT

THE SUN CREPT SLOWLY into the sky, bathing the terrain stretching out beneath the plane's wings in soft morning light. We'd been flying over the flat, brown plains in comfortable silence for hours.

'Hang on,' John spoke suddenly into his headset mic, dropping a wing to dive the plane.

As the plane descended, my stomach lifted and I became light in my seat. We were plummeting with ridiculous speed at an angle that was clearly going to miss the brown strip of ground that indicated the cattle station's runway. I held onto the handle above the window with one hand and gripped my leg with the other as the ground raced towards us uncomfortably quickly.

Kangaroos scattered into the trees, bouncing away at incredible speed. Seconds before impact, John pulled back on the stick and my bum sank into the seat as we swept back up into the clear sky. I let out a gasp of air before speaking shakily into my headset.

'Hah, ah, yeah. I thought you were going to crash there,

mate,' my voice crackled, filtered through the headset speakers.

'Crash?' he echoed, surprised. 'Nah, mate. That was a fly-by to scare the roos off the runway. We'll land her on the next pass.'

A few minutes later we landed on the biggest cattle station I'd ever heard of, let alone been to. The ranch was the size of a small country, and home to around 40,000 Brahman cattle. The cattle barely had any contact with humans, and so were essentially wild.

As we walked towards a small collection of wooden buildings, we were greeted with nods from the station workers. After a hot meal, I settled into my little room, throwing my bag into a corner and bouncing onto a squeaky mattress.

I fell into a deep sleep, ignorant of the morning ahead.

Wild Brahman will either run from you or run at you. If you don't learn to read the different signs quickly, you're as good as three backward rolls and a mouthful of dust. That's if you're lucky. It's broken bones or worse if you're not. The men and women who work the stock in the Outback are called 'ringers'. Seeing two ringers skittled by raging cows had confirmed I'd need to be quick on my feet to survive here.

That morning, the first thing I noticed was a dust cloud on the horizon. Next, I heard the staccato whumping of helicopters. Finally, there came the thundering of hooves, as thousands of cattle ran towards the yards, herded by helicopters above and horsemen on the ground.

The team ran them into a round holding pen the size of a football field. Once they were inside, we headed in on foot to push the cattle into smaller pens. We walked in a line about 10 metres apart, arms out wide as we faced down the mob. The animals circled and pushed each other like a school of fish herded by whistling dolphins. They kicked up dust that thickened in the air until I could barely make out the men on either side of me. The cattle were galloping grey silhouettes in the thick dust cloud.

I looked to my left to check that I was moving in line with the man beside me. When I returned my gaze to the mob, one of the silhouettes was charging me from the haze. I leapt to the side, and the cow's horns missed me by inches.

I looked to my right, and a bearded man with a cowboy hat grinned at me before sidestepping as another cow broke from the mob and charged him. The two cows were now pacing up and down behind us, throwing their heads. I looked back at them nervously, and then heard a warning whistle. I turned again to see another cow galloping towards me, her head down, hooves pounding the dust. I danced away at the last second, thankful for my years of rugby training. Now there were three behind us and thousands in front. One of the cows behind started charging the man to my left.

'Hey! Behind!' I called.

He turned and leapt to the side as she rushed back into the circling mob. The stranger gave me a nod of thanks.

I lost track of the minutes as I coughed in the dust and dodged raging cattle. Finally, we had enough of them in the smaller pens and I could leave the enormous holding pen. People pay good money to see a rodeo, and here we were in the middle of nowhere doing it for free. Well, at least I was, being a student.

The mayhem had left me caked with a thick layer of dust. My nostrils were clogged, and my throat burned.

Before I could recover, we were moving again, this time herding the cattle down the fenced narrow races to the smaller pens near the vet crush so they could be pregnancy checked.

John put his arm up the cows' backsides and felt for a foetus, or lack thereof. The rectal wall is thin, so a vet can easily palpate the uterus, which sits directly below. They can then give an estimate of how many months along the foetus is, or whether the cow is 'empty'.

From time to time I had a go and the ringers and John grinned as I tried to figure out what was going on in there. Eventually, with practice, my foetal age estimates got closer and closer to John's.

Sometimes a stubborn cow wouldn't move from a pen, at which point a surprising, if not questionable, tactic would be employed. Someone would leap into the pen and run past the angry ruminant, tempting the difficult bovine to chase them towards the open gate. Then the decoy would leap the fence at the last second, leaving the cow to run on through the gateway. They called this high-risk strategy 'clowning'.

Eventually, it was my turn to play rodeo clown. One big cow had decided she wouldn't budge from the round pen and move down the chute to be pregnancy checked. A young rooster from the UK, Jack, was working the pen, and he called out for a hand. John decided that, as I was a rugby player, it was only logical that I should assist.

The round pen is a central hub that allows cattle to be drafted off into different pens as they move through the yards. The worker pulls gates open and shut to get the cattle to move accordingly. It is a dangerous job, as the worker has to be standing in the pen with the cattle the entire time.

Jack had been battling with the angry cow, which seemed more interested in killing him than moving on from the pen, for a few minutes before he called out for help. He had been flipped over her back once already. Panting and covered in dust, he didn't seem keen on getting back in. Lines of darkened dust streaked his face, marking the tracks in which his sweat had run. A dirty drip hung from the bottom of his chin.

'Give us a hand and pop in that pen there and get her going — she's a fiery old devil!' Jack warned, bending to wash the dust from his eyes with his water bottle. He pointed to a tree behind the fence on the opposite side of the pen. 'That's your best line, I'd say.'

The cow was standing near the fence rails on the opposite side, facing Jack. Her head was down, and she was huffing angrily, clearly keen to finish what she'd started. I did a quick calculation in my head: it resulted in guaranteed contact with the 700-kilogram beast. Jack was now blinking blindly; he'd accidentally washed more dust into his eyes. I decided to make my own plan.

'Tell you what, Jack,' I said, pointing to another spot, 'I'll aim for that point next to the gate.' It was about half the distance he'd originally suggested for my run. He finally blinked the last of the dirt from his eyes and looked up. He wasn't too pleased with my compromise but shrugged in agreement. With no small degree of trepidation, I climbed to the top of the 2.5-metre-high rails and swung my legs over to sit facing my fate. By now the other ringers were leaning over the rails, sensing a show. The massive cow began trotting back and forth, throwing her head and frothing at the mouth in rage.

Taking a deep breath, I slid off the fence into the pen. The cow didn't stop to blink. As soon as my feet hit the dirt, the massive creature turned and accelerated at me at an astonishing speed. The extra time I had assumed I would get from her taking a moment to attack never eventuated. I turned and ran back up the fence. The cow slid to a stop in front of me, glaring up her challenge.

'Get down, ya pussy!' John had joined the spectators. 'Monkeys hang on rails; men get in the pen! You're a full-back for God's sake, you should be *fast*.'

I now regretted telling him my position on the rugby field,

or that I played the blasted sport at all. Sweat rolled down my face. The cow trotted a full circle, then lowered her head and pawed the ground, kicking dust back with her front foot, something I'd thought only happened in cartoons.

'Five years at vet school for nothing!' John jeered from the peanut gallery.

I couldn't take it anymore — I leapt from the fence and ran directly at the cow. She put her head down as the game of cow-and-chicken commenced. The distance closed rapidly as she barrelled towards me, her hooves hammering the dirt. Ten metres . . . 5 metres . . . *2 metres* — we were about to collide. She dipped her head and closed her eyes, readying for impact.

Time stood still.

Now.

I pushed off my toe, sidestepping. A rush of wind hit me as she swept past, far closer than I would have liked.

The men whooped and roared from the fence. I felt triumphant — until I turned to see that she had wheeled around for a second charge. Flat-footed and panicking, I slipped in the dust as I tried to run. My hands touched the ground, just keeping me on my feet, as my heart leapt into my throat.

Someone shouted at me, 'Move!' The laughter had died as the ringers saw I was about to be flattened. I leaned forward and sprinted for the fence, running faster than ever. In a flash, she was behind me, hooves thundering, her hot breath on the back of my legs. She was going to kill me. But it was there — the precious fence, my only hope.

I jumped high. A split second later the cow's head slammed inches below my feet, gonging the rails like a giant bell.

My waist hit the top rail and I flipped. My body somersaulted, twisting one-eighty, before miraculously righting itself to bring me in to land squarely on my feet on the other side. I'd landed facing back at the pen. I looked around, confused. John and the other ringers were staring at me, astonished.

The cow ran out of the pen and trotted into the vet race.

'Bloody hell, that was close,' John said. 'I didn't know you could do a rodeo flip.'

My hands were shaking as I picked up my hat and dusted it off. A few of the workers slapped me on the back as they made their way back to their spots in the yards. John looked at me curiously before following.

I stood for a moment, then nodded once. I will never do that again.

Five long days of working from dawn to sunset later, we refuelled the plane and took off for our next stop. I shifted uncomfortably in the little cockpit seat. A series of angry boils had appeared down the outside of my leg, the result of days on end in the dust and heat. The red bulges stung when I knocked them; I dreaded the moment I would need to lance them with one of the large needles in John's kit. I finally got comfortable and took the chance for some precious rest.

I snapped awake, my head lolling to the side as John banked the plane hard. He was sweeping yet another remote airstrip. The knowledge that this wasn't a manic landing attempt made the event less stressful this time. We pulled around again, and John lowered the flaps, dropping our air speed for a smooth touchdown.

This time we landed near a jumble of red rocks, scattered like a giant's discarded toys. There were only two buildings near the airstrip: an old, splintering stable, and a janky wooden structure that could have been a motel. There were no roads to speak of. It looked as though the only access to this place was by horseback, four-wheel-drive or aeroplane.

John cut the ignition and the engine sputtered to a stop. He pulled off his headset, signalling to me to do the same. I hastily struggled out of my jacket; the cockpit had scarcely taken a minute to become stiflingly hot now that we were on the ground.

'We won't be here long,' he told me. 'A ringer thinks his horse has broken her leg. There's already a vet here, but he wants a second opinion.'

He pointed to a group of stockmen gathered near the stables, some on horseback, others sitting under the shade of a lonely gum tree. 'Go ahead and take a look. I'll be over there in a bit.'

After collecting John's kit from the back, I made my way across the airstrip to where the men waited. My boots kicked up little puffs of dust as I trudged towards them. It was a cloudless day, and mercilessly hot without a breeze. By the time I had finished the short walk, sweat had beaded on my face. A tall, wiry man who was holding his injured horse on a lead rope turned to regard me as I approached, his expression darkening beneath his hat. 'Where's John?'

No small talk, then.

'He's on his way,' I explained, trying to keep my voice firm. He watched me coolly for a long moment, then stepped back to allow me to inspect his sleek bay mare. Her widened eyes showed her agitation, and her dark mane flicked as she tossed her head. She held her front-right leg up, with just the tip of the hoof gingerly brushing the ground.

Then I noticed a young vet among the group, her kit at her feet. There was an unmistakable look of irritation on her face. I hadn't noticed her before beneath her wide-brimmed leather hat.

The man spoke again. 'What do you think?'

The question hung there. A weighty thing, dangling between me and the stockmen.

I moved closer and eyed the injured leg, the mare moving her shoulder and the lower leg bent unnaturally. It was clearly broken. Most likely a clean, complete fracture of her cannon bone, a long bone below a horse's carpal joint in the forelimb, or tarsal joint in the hindlimb. It's a common bone for horses to fracture, as it takes a lot of force.

'It's broken,' I told him.

The man rubbed his brow, wincing.

'He's right, unfortunately.' John's arrival was timely.

The man rubbed his mare's neck gently, speaking to her quietly. After a long moment, he turned and nodded once to John. He knew what this meant.

By the time we left the group the sun had dropped, a deep blood orange hanging low on the horizon. The men had collected spades to dig her grave. I didn't envy them; the ground was like concrete.

I was sure they didn't envy me either. I had given her that very final injection. It wasn't the first time I had done it, but so far it was my most difficult euthanasia. She had wobbled once, then crashed to the ground. John had been in front of her, leaning back hard on her lead rope as she fell, pulling her head forward to stop it from hitting the packed earth. The man had watched me, his eyes far away, as I listened with my stethoscope to her heart's last thuds. When it stopped, I rose and told him that she was gone.

In the brief weeks I had been riding Tucker, I'd caught a glimpse of the type of bond that can grow between a person and their horse. But it wasn't until I saw the man's crestfallen face that I understood how deep that bond could go.

We boarded the plane in silence and flew back to town one last time.

John's pen poised over my clinical assessment sheet. It was my last afternoon at the clinic before I flew back to New Zealand.

'Animal handling . . .' he read aloud. His marker hovered over the unsatisfactory box, then drifted one box over to marginal. He ticked it.

'Marginal?' I complained. 'I got into a pen and went toe-to-toe with a seven hundred-kilogram wild cow!'

'Yeah, and she nearly ran you down,' he retorted.

I let out an exasperated breath as he meandered down to the next line. Professionalism. He ticked 'marginal' once again.

'When you first arrived here, I thought you were a dud. But you got a bit better towards the end,' he explained.

I looked up at the walls as if I could rally support from the dosing charts and pet-food posters.

'John, this counts towards my final grade,' I protested. 'I've cleaned shit off your gear every day for the last month, for crying out loud!'

'Did I ask you to do that?'

'Yes, you bloody well did!'

'Exactly. I shouldn't need to ask. You should just do it. You're too slow and you lean on fences. Keep going the way you are, and you'll waste away like an old granny.'

I dragged my hands through my hair, defeated.

John dropped the pen and regarded me seriously. 'This is for your own good, you know. That other student in there,' he thrust a thumb over his shoulder towards the next room. 'I'm not going to waste time bollocking him. But you . . .' he paused, watching me.

I stared back at him uncomprehendingly. He seemed to be gearing up to pay me a compliment. I'd never heard him compliment anyone, so I was both confused and intrigued. 'There's potential,' he finished.

I was too surprised to answer, so John returned his

attention to the page. His pen trailed down the paper, relentlessly ticking the 'marginal' boxes. There was a moment when it drifted across to satisfactory, and even a precious second where I saw him consider the 'good' box. But in a flash it was gone as he shook his head and returned to his barrage on my grades.

As I trudged to the bus holding my assessment in a sealed envelope, I glanced down at the bandages on my leg, the result of my assault on the boils the night before. I would need to change them soon.

I shook my head. I had bigger things than a single assessment to worry about. My final exams were looming. One last hurdle before freedom. Before income. Before real adult life began. It was time to fly away from the biting bugs, crocodiles, boils and charging cattle.

At least, for now.

CHAPTER EIGHT

INTO THE WORLD

The cat gasps for air and struggles violently against you. What do you do next?

I WAS KILLING THE CAT. If the cat died, I failed the exam. It was as simple as that. It would mean a whole summer of studying while my friends celebrated graduating. Not to mention I would lose the job I was supposed to be starting in a month's time.

I had been dumbfounded by the job offers that had come in the weeks following John's month-long assault on my work ethic, upbringing, intellect, sports team preferences and personality in general. I'd operated on autopilot, moving cattle, filling buckets with warm water, setting gear out for the vets, cleaning their trucks. I memorised the equipment they needed on each call, where they had stored the assorted pieces in their truck, then pulled them out before John could shout at me. Then I'd remember he wasn't there. The vets had thrown me disbelieving looks as I hustled about performing tasks.

Eventually, I'd decided to accept a job in Canterbury. It was close to home, and Don had been offered a job there, too. It was a large clinic in the countryside, focused mainly on dairy farms, although there was a small companion-animal clinic attached. Don and I would have similar roles, taking on the 'grunt work' of dairy vetting, and dabbling in the small-animal clinic whenever someone wandered in with a pooch or cat. I preferred the physical challenge and to be out on farms in the fresh air, so I'd found myself gravitating towards farm vet work in my last few years at university.

The computer-simulation cat had been hit by a car and was now breathing in short, rapid breaths. I had already given it some pain relief and a mild sedative, but trying to do an X-ray had clearly been a mistake. Giving it oxygen with a mask had made things worse, too. I guessed that I had one more try before the blasted thing died and my summer was over. My mouse drifted over the six options like a little white fly unsure of where to land.

I looked across at Don. He seemed calm. I heard sobbing from behind me. I turned in my chair to see a girl with her face in her hands. Her back was shaking as she cried. Her cat must have died.

I clicked 'put the cat in an oxygen cage', and held my breath. I was the one needing oxygen. The screen flicked to the next page.

The cat seems to settle, its breathing improves.

I let out my breath, a long hiss of air. I was finally helping this pixelated minx. I heard another burst of sobbing from the far side of the room as the software claimed another victim. The program finally let me take an X-ray, and I realised the cat had air in its chest space, a condition called a pneumothorax. I selected 'perform a chest tap', which meant I would put a needle into the chest space and suck the air out of this cyber cat. It hypothetically recovered, and I finally finished the last section of the exam.

A great heaviness fell from me as I rose from my chair. I pushed open the exam room door to see Don waiting for me in the hallway, one straw hat on his head, another in his hands.

He raised an eyebrow as he stuck the hat on my head.

'Well, the animals lived, at least,' I shrugged.

Don cheered. 'We did it!'

We ran down the hall and across the quad towards a waiting bus. A smattering of classmates stood around it, drinking beers and chatting. Pepper and Olive were among them, waving us in. The others were still trickling out from the exam building, a range of expressions on their faces. Some looked shaken, but for the most part I saw relief. The great burden we had been carrying for months was finally lifting.

We climbed aboard and the singing began. Our victory tour was under way. That night, our dreary little university town was the site of our own parade. We were the champions.

Two days later, Don and I were walking down to a remote beach. Don was carrying a shovel over one shoulder, and I had my surfboard tucked under my arm. Little rocky pinnacles dotted the horizon, poking up from the ocean like the teeth of a senile crocodile. We had driven to the Coromandel, and it was spectacular.

Don stopped and dug his toes into the sand. 'Pretty sure it's here somewhere . . . OUCH!' He danced back from the spot, then smiled in triumph. 'Try that.'

As I tentatively dug my toes down into the sand, boiling-hot water touched my foot. I snapped it back and looked up at Don. 'It's real!'

We began digging. Scalding water began to fill the hole, and I had to stop using my hands and let Don carry on with the shovel. After 10 minutes we had a decent-sized hole, but the water was too hot to sit in, so we created a sand channel to let water from the incoming tide rush into the hole, bringing it down to a more reasonable temperature.

We eased ourselves in, and I lay back in our sandy hot tub, feeling the last remnants of exam stress soak away. Gulls dived and soared in the sea breeze.

'It doesn't get much better than this, Don,' I announced.

Don nudged my leg. 'You're wrong,' he said.

Two summer-tanned women in bikinis were walking towards our little sand spa. Don's mouth was hanging open slightly. I kicked him back.

'Don't stare, you idiot,' I muttered.

Don kicked me again. 'You're the one staring!'

Before I could land a final kick, they stood over us. One

was tall and blonde, the other was shorter, with dark wavy hair. She looked athletic, the type of woman who could pass a rugby ball hard enough to sting your hands.

Don and I must have looked like two stunned mullets lying in a puddle, because a hint of amusement touched the blonde woman's eyes. 'How do you find the hot water?' she asked us, rounding out the word 'hoew'.

Don and I both tried to answer at the same time, then stopped. Then we tried again, our voices muddling together. Finally, I let Don explain. He had found the water first and it was only fair.

'You just dig around and test the water. But you shouldn't dig with your hands, because you'll burn them like this guy did,' he finished, gesturing at me with an air of superiority.

'Oh no, are your hands okay?' the shorter girl asked me with a look of concern.

A disgruntled look flashed across Don's face as the girls' attention shifted to me.

'Well . . . they are still a little sore . . .' I said. 'But I'm fine.' The taller of the two had begun gazing down the beach, growing bored, so I hastily pressed on. 'You're welcome to join us. It would save you a lot of digging . . .'

To my surprise, they squeezed in between us. Don looked as though he'd just won the lottery. I suspect my face didn't look much different. He started to talk to the blonde girl, who had nestled in beside him.

The dark-haired girl turned to face me. 'I'm Amber.' She grasped my hand gently, giving it a light squeeze. The sides of our bodies were pressed together as we lay in the warm water.

'Marcus.' I grinned, trying my best to keep my smile from extending to my ears. 'Are you Canadian?' I asked.

'We sure are,' she replied. She returned my smile and then took my hand once more, this time not letting go. My throat tightened and I swallowed dryly. 'This is my sister, Flor.'

Flor looked up from her conversation with Don and scrunched her eyes at me warmly. Don, sitting behind her, looked as though he might need to be tethered to a rock to keep from floating away to join the gulls.

I was 23 and had never been in love, but that was about to change. Amber was about to capture my heart in a way only first love can. The feeling was so powerful it was shocking — a gut-wrenching, ecstatic bliss, the type of reckless love that can only be felt by someone who's never been heartbroken. A blind and dazed perfect folly. But it wouldn't happen without risk: without taking a great leap of faith that could well leave me rejected and embarrassed.

The four of us spent the next few days visiting beaches and bays, climbing hills, and going out for drinks and meals. Amber and I awkwardly courted while Don and Flor exchanged amused glances.

Two weeks later, I hugged Amber goodbye. It felt stiff, almost uncomfortable. Next to me, Don gave Flor a more relaxed embrace. A voice rang out from the airport speakers, reminding us that their flight was boarding soon. I said a few mechanical things about having a safe flight, and before I knew it she was walking away.

I watched her wend her way between the ropes towards the security checkpoint. What had I done? She was leaving with no idea how I felt towards her because I'd never once told her. The chances of me ever meeting her again were slim to none: she was off to Australia, then back home. Ten thousand miles away.

Don pressed his lips together, looking down. We turned and began to walk away.

'Don, I should have said something,' I said, my voice cracking with despair.

'Yes, you should have,' he said.

There was a long pause, then I stopped. Don looked up at me.

'I could go back?' It was beginning to feel like a movie cliché.

Don looked over at Amber and Flor who were nearing the front of the line, then back to me. A wild grin spread across his face. 'Go,' he said. I was frozen on the spot. 'Go. Go!'

A tightness filled my chest, as if a huge air bubble was rising to sit at the base of my throat. Don stared at me wide-eyed, urging me forward.

'I'm going,' I declared. Don started pogo jumping with excitement. I turned and began to run. Passengers gazed at me as I shot past them, beelining for the security checkpoint. Amber was just about to put her bag down on the conveyor belt.

'Amber!' I called.

She stopped midway through lifting her bag and looked over at me, surprised.

I didn't have a plan.

'Can you come here?' I asked, out of breath from my dash.

Her sister grinned as Amber passed her the bag and began to wind her way back out from the security point. It took a painfully long time for her to zigzag her way back to me. Finally, she stood in front of me.

I took a deep breath. 'I've waited to meet a woman like you for a really long time.' The words tumbled from me. 'I know we didn't spend much time together, but, well, I am so glad I met you, you're sweet and kind and fun and gorgeous...'

I met her eyes, they were intense, fixed on mine. Then her smile danced up to play in them.

'I truly hope we meet again, Amber,' I told her, gravely.

'Me, too,' she agreed. 'Who knows what will happen . . . ?' She pulled me in. This time we held each other long and tight. I could feel her softness, her warmth, her breath.

Finally, we parted, and she went to join her sister and board her flight as I wandered back to Don.

I felt like I'd just kicked the winning goal for the All Blacks at the Rugby World Cup. But I still had enough sense to make sure we got out of sight of them before we started our victorious jig, Don spinning me around and hooting.

To my delight, Amber messaged me three weeks later to say she was coming back to New Zealand.

University was over, and a new life had begun.

CHAPTER NINE

PIGOCALYPSE

THE NEEDLE ON THE SPEEDOMETER vibrated at the 90-kilometres-per-hour line as I rattled down a backcountry road. A ute overtook me, the sheepdogs watching me from the back as it passed, their fur blustering in the wind. Being the newest vet to the clinic meant I got the oldest truck, in this case the 'Grey Rattler'. Other vets would have to leave before I was promoted to something with cruise control, Bluetooth or, better still, heated seats.

I was nervous. It was my first weekend on call, the first real test of my ability to deal with cases on my own. We mostly saw dairy cows during the week; however, already this weekend I had been called to see an alpaca, a horse and a goat, and I had even stitched up a hunting dog that had been gored by a boar.

You'd think this would have been stressful, but it hadn't been, because in between calls I'd been going to see Amber. She had been back in New Zealand for a month, and this was our last week together. We'd fallen in love fast, and the world outside of her had shrunk to nothing. As I made my way to the call-out, I couldn't have summoned a wisp of anxiety if I'd tried.

Besides, even if I hadn't been a love-intoxicated frolicker, I could have spent 100 years fretting over different scenarios and *still* not have come up with the mess I was driving towards.

When I first received the text message, I thought the office girls had got hold of the on-call service and were playing a prank.

The stressed tone of the pig farmer on the phone told me otherwise. This was real.

The truck clunked loudly as I lurched over a bump in the road. I couldn't complain about my rattly truck, however — I was lucky to have been given another vehicle after what had happened to the previous one a few weeks earlier.

I had been driving home from work, my mind on a million different things at once as I'd flown down the highway. I had crossed the train tracks, pulled around a corner, and glanced down as my beeper went off on the centre console. I hadn't even had a chance to look back up before—

BANG!

The airbag exploded in my face and the car jolted violently, the shock vibrating through my body as it skidded off the road and lurched to a stop. I got out to check the damage: the front wheel on the driver's side was smashed, as was the side of the car. I turned to see what I had hit. A half-wrecked car sat in the middle of the road, where it had been waiting to turn when I hit it from behind. A woman was still inside.

As I fumbled for what to do next, one of the senior vets drove up and pulled over. Together we crossed the road to the woman's car. I could see she was conscious, but stunned. I opened the door.

'Can you move?' I asked. My colleague began stopping the traffic.

She nodded and climbed, trembling, from the wreck. I helped her from the highway and sat her down on the side of the road. I struggled to speak. What could I say? Sorry that I nearly killed you? She had whiplash, but otherwise seemed to be okay.

It wasn't long before two fire engines arrived, then an ambulance, then two police cars. The highway was a dazzle of flashing lights and uniformed men and women hurrying across the shrapnel-covered asphalt. I felt sick as I explained what had happened to the police officer. It felt like an eternity before I was headed home, now in the passenger seat of my workmate's ute.

When we'd been cautioned in class about the alarming number of vets who got into car wrecks in their first year of practice, I'd thought: not me. *I'm* a good driver. I had never had a crash before, and I didn't plan to now. I'd dismissed the warning and allowed it to float away to join the other space junk in my mind's outer orbit. I assumed the need to exercise extra care while driving didn't apply to me.

Now, I winced at the painful lesson I'd learned. All I could do was thank God that no one had been seriously hurt. I shook the memory from my mind: I was at the farm, and it was time to focus.

When I pulled into the property, I was met with chaos. Fences were trampled. Pigs were scattered across the paddock, some lying down panting, others huddled in corners. One lay in the middle of the track ahead of me, clearly dead. Some had minor lacerations. One large sow had blood coming from her nose.

The farmer drove up in his ute, his face etched with tension. He answered my question before it had left my lips.

'I was feeding out, and then I looked up and couldn't believe my eyes. A hot-air balloon. The guy must have miscalculated his landing, I don't know.' He shook his head, then went on. 'The balloon came straight at us, drifting in the wind. It was right above us when he blasted the whisper burner. It sounded like a flame thrower — the pigs went berserk.'

He gestured to the mayhem around us. 'They stampeded, wrecked the fences, ran into each other . . . Some of them might even be off the property now, I'm not sure. If they get scared enough, they can die from a heart attack. Like she did.' He pointed to the pig on the track. 'I think she's the only one that has died, so far at least. The one in the hedge over there might be close.'

In the nearby hedgerow a pink creature was lying on its side, panting. What the hell do I do? The silence stretched. This was the moment when I came up with some genius plan of attack and fixed everything, right? I thought back to my university courses on pigs. All that I found was a collection of useless facts about pig growth rates and sow-crate dimensions. Clearly, I was going to have to make this one up as I went along.

'Shall we take a drive so I can get a full idea of what's going on?' I suggested. 'We can see if any of them need treatment.'

He nodded in agreement. 'I will need a report from you to send to the insurance company.'

Well, it was a start. The only problem was that I had no idea how I would catch any of them, let alone treat them. I climbed onto the flat-bed of his ute, and he drove me on a slow expedition across the farm.

He pulled over in front of one of the pens and leaned out the window. Most of the pigs were standing in small groups, but a few stood alone, staring into space. They were oddly quiet. One was lying down, panting, her eyes closed. I jotted down some notes. I took a closer look at one, and saw that dark bruising rimmed her eye. She must have run into something in the chaos.

The next pen was in a similar state; the only pig with obvious injuries was one with some minor cuts. She must have got caught running through the fence. Getting hold of her to clean the wounds would have been ideal, but the fences were broken and there was no way to pen her up.

The pigs were also so stressed that any attempt to handle them could bring on heart failure and kill them.

I recalled a pig's piercing squeals as I caught it with a snare during a handling lab at university. I considered the long pole in my truck with a syringe attached to the end. I could get the pole syringe and knock her out with a tranquiliser? No . . . the wounds were too minor to justify that.

How can it be that some animals become so frightened that they die? It can happen to sheep harried by dogs, and birds, too. You would think thousands of years of natural selection would have removed such a trait. At university they had used words like 'shock' and 'stress'. In some animals, the heart rate and blood pressure can climb so high from fright that it kills them.

These poor animals would have looked up to see a fire-blowing 'dragon' coming to eat them. No wonder they had panicked. Pigs are of similar intelligence to dogs. These pigs were smart enough to understand something unusual and threatening was happening, but were not able to comprehend what it was.

This was a free-range farm. The pigs had space to walk around their paddocks, root about the ground, socialise and, well, be pigs. I will never forget the pleading eyes of the sows I had once seen on a class farm visit. They had stared up at me helplessly from row after row of cramped pens called sow stalls. They had been so restricted in the narrow spaces that they couldn't even turn around. All they could do was move half a metre forward or back. The stalls were preferred by farmers because they reduced piglet losses, but they were terrible for the sows. I recall thinking that we treat prisoners with more decency. Thankfully, sow stalls are now banned in New Zealand and many other countries.

We continued along the farm track. The other pigs were in varying states of distress, and I recorded a few more minor injuries. Another pig was lying dead in her pen. I decided it would be best to give the pig in the hedge time and space to calm down. Hopefully, she would move out on her own.

Once we got back to the entrance, I climbed off the back of the ute and walked up to the driver's window. 'I think the only thing we can do right now is give them some space. From what I saw the scrapes on that sow looked minor. If there are any that you're worried about still, you could pen them up later this evening and I can come back and clean them up.'

'That sounds good to me,' he said.

'I'll have the report to you in the next few days,' I told him.

I took a final look at the broken fences; the poor chap had a lot of work ahead of him. I climbed back into the Grey Rattler and made my way back to Amber. It was time to say goodbye.

As a distraction, I pictured my workmates' faces the next day when I told them the story of the pigs. They'd love it. Then again, maybe they wouldn't believe me and think it was just a load of hot air.

CHAPTER TEN

FART & PIT

THINGS WERE FINALLY STARTING to make sense. If an old cat comes in that's losing weight and 'not themself', first check the teeth to rule out dental disease. If it's not a dental issue, chances are it's going to be a thyroid problem, kidney failure or maybe diabetes. Of course, it could be something else, but I had begun to understand that the quickest and cheapest route was to rule out the common problems first, thereby saving the owner time and expense.

Mrs Thatcher watched as I listened to Belle's heart. She patted her neat grey hair, and then clasped her hands in her lap. Belle was a pretty, long-haired cat with grey fur and a flat face. Her heartbeat was loud and bounding. It was unusually fast. I ran my fingers down the front of her neck, below her chin, feeling either side of Belle's trachea to try to detect an abnormally large thyroid gland. I couldn't feel one. I frowned, concentrating. Mrs Thatcher leaned close and murmured soothing words to her beloved cat.

A distracting pain had been niggling at me all morning, an odd, empty feeling pushing up at the base of my heart.

Amber had flown out to Thailand the night before. Saying goodbye to her had felt like having an organ removed. Something vital to my every breath was missing. I couldn't believe she was gone.

'Is something wrong?' Mrs Thatcher asked. Whether it was my own pain she detected or whether she suspected a thyroid problem in Belle, I couldn't say.

'I'm not entirely sure yet, but I am wondering if she might have a thyroid issue. Her heart is racing and . . .' I watched Belle closely: she was hyperactive, looking around the room, her head bobbing and weaving. 'And I think it would be wise to take a blood sample, to check her thyroid levels. We can also look at some other things that can tell us about her liver and kidneys, as well as her blood sugar.'

'Do whatever you need to,' she said.

I left the room and returned moments later with Sarah, one of the nurses. Sarah tilted the cat's head back so I could clip away the fur over the neck, exposing the skin over the jugular vein. I wiped firmly down Belle's neck with a cotton bud wet with methylated spirits, then pressed my thumb down low on the neck, raising the vein. It was only a few millimetres wide, and it was important the cat didn't move as I approached with the needle. I homed in on the spot, my vision narrowed, all my concentration focused. The needle was just an inch from the skin when a long, melancholic note trumpeted into the silence. I startled. We all did.

My back-end emission was so resounding that it was impossible to deny. It seemed to ask a question, the note rising a touch at the end. Even the cat looked offended. The needle was now in the cat's neck. The only problem was that the cat now vibrated as Sarah tried to contain her laughter, little bursts of air snorting from her nose, her eyes scrunched closed, her face red. Fortunately, I was also bobbing with stifled laughter, and miraculously keeping in time with the cat. Belle was so perplexed that she just stared out into space as the blood flowed easily into the syringe.

I glanced over at Mrs Thatcher, clearly a woman of discipline, but even her smirk could not be disguised. I withdrew the needle from the remarkably compliant cat and transferred the blood into a sample tube. Tears were now running down Sarah's face.

I attempted to speak to Mrs Thatcher.

'Mrs Thatcher, we—' It was hopeless: I couldn't contain myself. Like something from a bad dream, my attempts to stifle my laughter had only squeezed it to a ridiculous pitch.

After a few deep breaths, I cleared my throat and tried again. 'We will run the sample and — and see what we — we can find . . .' My voice sounded as though I'd swallowed helium.

Sarah and I made a hasty exit, leaving the perplexed puss and her stunned owner behind. When Mrs Thatcher had put Belle back in her carrier and approached the counter to pay, for once I had nothing to say as I keyed numbers into the card reader. A moment before, Sarah had disappeared into the back office and now an explosion of laughter burst from behind us, the hoots echoing out to fill the reception area. Mrs Thatcher tactfully hid another smile behind her hand as I took her card and ran it.

'I'll call you with the results. Err . . . Have a lovely day . . . It looks beautiful outside,' I finished up awkwardly.

'Thank you. It'll be nice to get out and enjoy some fresh air,' she replied levelly, as she punched her PIN number into the pad on the card reader.

Well played, Thatcher.

Her cane clicked away as she exited the building through the automatic doors, Belle's cage in hand.

I turned to the open office door, readying myself for what was to come. As I walked in, I saw every office chair was facing me. Then my co-workers stood and clapped.

A few days later I called Mrs Thatcher with the results. Belle's thyroxine levels were high, and she needed treatment. The excess thyroxine meant that her metabolism was in overdrive, and she couldn't eat enough to keep up. This caused her to lose weight despite having a ravenous appetite.

There was the option for Belle to go to a clinic and have radiation treatment to reduce the size of her thyroid gland, and, as a result, the amount of thyroxine produced. However, Belle was old, and after I explained the cost and risks to her, Mrs Thatcher opted for daily pills.

As I hung up the phone, one of my colleagues spoke without looking up from his paperwork. 'That poor old lady is still breathing, then? The miracles I see in practice never cease to amaze me.'

The comments about experimental noxious gas treatments, and the unregistered use of potent sedatives on patients *and* clients, had finally reduced to a trickle.

'Oh yes,' I replied tartly, 'and from what I hear, her asthma has cleared up: a magic cure, the doctors say.'

'I think I'd prefer asthma,' he shot back.

At that moment, Richard, our boss, walked into the office. 'The Donaldsons have a situation,' he said to me. 'I told them you'd be there in ten minutes. One of their workers, Dylan, will meet you at the shed.'

I sped past the macrocarpa hedges that lined the country road. An emergency didn't give a vet permission to speed, but I put my foot down a little more anyway. The Grey Rattler had been replaced by a decent machine with real power. It could surge through rivers and plough through a muddy paddock as if it were an autumn puddle.

Richard had given me the few details he had as I grabbed my overalls and ran for the truck. A cow had half-fallen into the centre pit in the Donaldsons' rotary dairy shed. She was halfway under a rail, her front end hanging down and her back still up in her milking bail.

Rotary sheds are circular, with cows standing in any given number of 'bails' around the outer edge of the circle. Their heads face the centre, and their tails and udders face back so that a milker can put milking cups on the teats for the cows to be milked.

Some rotary sheds, like this one, had a deep concrete pit in the centre. The circular pit was about 8 metres across, and 3.5 metres deep. It was supposed to be impossible for a cow to get through the rails to the pit, but this one had been determined. She had forced her head and two front legs between the rails and partially fallen in. Only her hips kept her wedged in place. Cows are not designed to dangle. She needed to be freed, and soon.

I pulled onto the gravel track leading up to the shed, lurching to a stop outside the shed door. I took the sedation medication from the back and was in the act of drawing some up when Dylan came out of the shed.

'She fell in,' Dylan told me. 'Looks as though she isn't hurt.' Then he added, sensing my question, 'Now, we have a bigger problem. Even if you can knock her out, the pit is ten feet deep . . .'

I followed him into the shed, and, sure enough, the cow was standing down in the pit, looking around idly, chewing her cud as if disappointed in the outcome of her acrobatic efforts. She was standing evenly on all four feet with barely a scratch on her. She walked a half-circle around the pit and, surprisingly, didn't limp at all. The shed was a spider's web of steel rails criss-crossed from the upper rim of the pit. She was thoroughly trapped.

Through the doors and across the yard I saw a telehandler constructing a nearby shed, its proboscis-like winch arm picking up a piece of sheet metal. I pointed to the man working the machine in the distance.

'Do you think that guy would help?' I asked. Dylan trotted off towards the work site to find out. In the meantime, I went back to the truck and assembled my pole syringe.

The pole syringe is made up of two long pieces of metal tubing that interlock, with a syringe attached to one end. Vets can use them to jab animals, usually with a sedative, from a distance. I locked the two pieces together, attached a needle to the end, then carefully drew up the sedation into the syringe. It was a ketamine-xylazine mix — powerful stuff.

One of my colleagues once pricked her finger with a needle after using it. She thought she would be fine, but phoned the clinic just to be safe. The manager had driven to the farm only to discover our colleague wasn't there. A little further down the road the manager found her asleep in her truck beside a river. She was lucky. She'd taken only a prick of sedative and was soon revived in hospital.

Now, as I walked back to the shed, carrying the loaded pole syringe safely away from my body, I saw the telehandler being driven over, Dylan alongside.

News of the bovine predicament had spread, and curious builders and farm staff were arriving to watch the drama. The spectators lined the upper rim of the pit as I climbed over the rails. I was now the day's entertainment.

The cow kept a wary eye on me as I hung off the wall and dropped into the pit, watched by a crowd dressed in an assortment of high-vis vests and overalls. It was dim down there. A farmworker passed down the loaded pole syringe.

There is an art to making a non-threatening walk towards livestock. I circled the pit without making eye contact with the cow. She let me get almost within striking distance before loping away, her hoofs clicking on the concrete as she ran around the edge ahead of me, stopping on the opposite side to look at me again. I cursed silently.

'She's on to you,' one of the onlookers goaded, his deep voice echoing in the pit. I was already regretting doing this with an audience.

I walked the other way, again not looking at the cow. This time, when I reached her flight distance, I was ready. As she turned to run, I dashed forward and lunged my spear out. The needle struck the back of her thigh, right on target, and the syringe, compressed by the impact, injected the drug into her muscle. She skipped a little at the jab, then continued her trot to the other side. My audience gave a half-enthused cheer, clearly disappointed that the chase had ended so soon and hadn't included the cow charging me.

By now the telehandler had pulled up and was parked in the entranceway to the shed, where the cows walked on and off the milking platform.

I called up to the winch operator, 'Can you bring it in?'

'I'll give it my best shot!' he shouted back over the thrum of the engine. 'It'll be tight!'

I leaned back against the wall and waited. I could see the cow was starting to hang her head a little. The drug was taking effect.

The winch operator pulled the massive vehicle further up to the milking bails, as close as he could. He pressed a button on his dash and the winch arm began to extend. He had found a miraculous gap between the rails and the milking units, and the arm cleared the space with inches to spare.

Finally, it stopped, the hook hanging right above the now-groggy cow. She took a few stumbling steps and knelt. Her bottom pointed defiantly in the air as she managed to stay standing on her wobbly back legs. At last, she settled and lay down, and soon she was fast asleep.

Dylan climbed into the pit with me. Together we pulled a sling under the cow's body, and then he signalled to the winch operator to lower the large metal hook. The chain rattled as it wobbled down to meet us. We attached the sling to the hook and gave the winch operator a thumbs-up.

He began to lift. The chain clanked as it took the cow's weight and became taut. We held our breath as she slowly lifted from the floor, her hooves dragging on the concrete as her weight aligned with the chain. Up and up she went, until she was almost touching the ceiling. Her legs and head hung limply. He carefully reversed the machine, and the cow cleared the rails. It was a tight squeeze, and just as it was starting to look as though she would fit, her leg hooked on a rail.

'Stop!' Dylan and I called out.

I climbed up the pit wall, and, avoiding standing directly beneath the 600-kilogram dangling cow, pushed her hoof and unhooked it from the rail. Finally, she was free and moving again. It was with huge relief we saw her lowered safely down into one of the milking bails.

The audience gave a more enthused cheer this time. The cow let out a soft, tired 'moo' as we untied her sling.

I made my way around to her back end and lifted her tail, prodding at the underside of it with the end of my finger. I was looking for the spot between the tail vertebrae to give her an injection of the reversal drug for the sedative. I had a smaller, more traditional syringe this time. I advanced the needle and, to my satisfaction, the clear liquid inside turned dark red as I hit the vein.

I injected it slowly, and then stood back. She jumped up within seconds, backed out of the milking bail, turned and trotted off to her paddock. The whole thing had taken only 20 minutes.

'I thought we would have to put her down.'

I turned at the sound of a new voice. It was the farm owner. My latex glove thwacked against my wrist as I pulled it off in preparation to shake his hand.

'I was nervous when your boss said a new vet was coming out, but you did a fine job here,' he said, giving me a respectful nod.

'I think it's this fella on the telehandler you should be

thanking,' I said, and the farm owner turned to shake the man's hand before shaking mine.

It had been a team effort, but nonetheless my chest puffed out a little. It had been a tense situation and I'd managed. As a new vet, making a good first impression with a farm owner never hurts.

CHAPTER ELEVEN

TIGER'S TOOTH

I GENTLY LIFTED the tomcat's big paw, idly stroking the leathery palm as I listened. I set my stethoscope back down on the table. His name was Tiger — an odd name for a black cat, but I had heard stranger. Tiger's owner, Thomas, sat patiently in the waiting room as we worked. Tiger's heartbeat had sounded slow but was otherwise normal. He was breathing long and deep. I was satisfied to see the sedation working perfectly.

Sarah met my eye as she finished positioning the X-ray machine. I gave her a thumbs-up and we left the room. The small grey remote she grasped trailed a coiled wire through the doorway and back to the machine.

'X-ray!' she called, then pressed the button firmly.

The result might have been an earth-shattering cannon explosion if I'd listened to the call of the military three years before. Back then, as I'd listlessly thumbed through a dreary, thick textbook on canine anatomy, I had heard the soldiers training nearby from my desk at university, and I'd toyed with the temptation to march from the campus over to the barracks to sign up. Running through a forest throwing grenades had a certain boredom-breaking appeal. I had wanted to hurl the textbook out of the window of the vet school tower's fifth floor and watch it flap down and splash into the pond below.

But I hadn't, so I was now met instead with a soft beep as the X-ray machine told us it was safe to return to the examination room.

I held the sleek, muscled animal as Sarah slid the X-ray plate out from under him.

A moment later I led Thomas to the computer to examine the black-and-white image. Tiger had stopped eating, and it seemed I had found the cause. I pointed to a large opaque oval high in his abdomen.

'See this here?' I asked. Thomas nodded, furrowing his brow as he followed my finger.

'That's his kidney. It's enlarged,' I said.

His frown deepened as he turned to look at me. 'What could cause that?' he asked solemnly.

I hesitated before answering. It was hard news to deliver, but was it not my job to be honest? Impartial? Tell things as they are? I cleared my throat. 'Well . . . I hate to say it, but it's likely a tumour on the kidney.'

The poor man's jaw went slack. 'Cancer?' He breathed the word. His pale-blue eyes glistened as they filled with tears. He blinked them away and took a deep breath before meeting my eyes once more. 'What's to be done, then?' he asked, forcing his voice to remain level.

'I'm sorry,' I began, in what I hoped was a comforting

tone, 'but I'm going to refer you to a vet down the road, Andy; he has much more experience with this type of thing than I do.'

I gazed out the window, watching Thomas carry Tiger out to the car now that he had recovered sufficiently from his sedation.

'Cancer?'

I jumped; Sarah had come to stand beside me.

'Nasty business,' I sighed. 'Damn shame that we don't have a cure.' As I glanced over at her, I saw on her face what might have been a question forming. Then it was gone.

'Go ahead, ask it,' I urged her. It was good for the nurses to feel free to ask questions.

She didn't speak right away. 'Well . . .' She hesitated as if reconsidering, then pressed on. 'How do you know it was cancer?'

It was an understandable question. Sarah was a good nurse, but she hadn't had those *years* of extra training that I'd had.

I bobbed my head patiently. 'That kidney was enormous. I really can't imagine what else it could be but a tumour.'

Sarah looked as though she was about to ask another question but stopped, instead sounding a hum of interest before disappearing to pack away the X-ray equipment.

A few days later, Thomas reappeared. He strode into the clinic, a grin spread across his wrinkled cheeks.

'Thomas?' I queried. Strange things, coping mechanisms. I made a mental note to watch a YouTube video on the matter.

'That I am! As surely as the sun shines — all that was wrong with Tiger was a rotten tooth!' he chirped.

I stared at him dumbly.

He continued, 'That old vet down the road looked at the X-ray and his eyeballs just about fell out! A normal tomcat's kidney he told me. Wasn't enlarged at all.'

Large male cats can have much bigger kidneys than other cats; I had no idea. I tried to stammer a reply, but Thomas had already spun on his happy heels and was heading out the door.

I was still standing there gazing out the window a minute after he had driven away. Maybe that's the end of it? I tried to console my deflated pride.

A moment later my phone vibrated. I pulled it out to read the message.

> I hear you caused quite an uproar at
> Andy's clinic today? ;)

It was my brother. How on earth did he know about this? He worked in marketing for a gym on the other side of the city for crying out loud . . .

'Who's that?!'

I just about leapt out of my surgery Crocs. 'Bloody hell,

Sarah, you need to stop doing that!' I scolded.

'I would have won twenty bucks, you know,' she continued as if she hadn't just blown my eardrums out. She waited for me to interrogate her but, seeing that I wasn't biting, pressed on anyway. 'Only, I couldn't find anyone to back your diagnosis.'

I didn't have anything to say, so I returned to my sullen gazing out the window.

'About that notorious kidney, that is,' she added, driving the point home.

There was another army base near the clinic. Maybe they would accept a failed vet?

As if reading my thoughts, Sarah relented and softened her tone. 'It happens to all the new grads who come through here. Then they realise they don't know anything, and — *poof!*' She flicked her fingers dramatically. 'It's all good.'

I couldn't decide which was worse: the revelation that I was ignorant, or the epiphany that I had been ignorant of my ignorance.

CHAPTER TWELVE

BLOAT

I SAT AT MY DESK and read the sentence in my cattle textbook for the fourth time. I still had no idea what it said. I was bored. We all were.

The dairy season was broken up into busy times and quiet times. The spring rush brought calvings, metabolic problems, down cows, sick calves, mastitis. Then de-budding calves, which was when we sedated calves and removed the horn buds to keep them from becoming dangerous to their herdmates and farmers. Then came treating metritis, infection of the uterus — a messy and stinky job. This led to pre-mating blood sampling and fertility treatment. Following this was early-pregnancy scanning, then a lull over Christmas before late-pregnancy scanning got under way.

When the cows got to the end of the milking season, around May, we would perform teat sealing, a fiddly job where we put a sealant into cows' teats to stop them getting infections while they were dried off and not milking. Getting the teat sealant into heifers was the hardest. The young, first-time-pregnant animals hadn't been handled much and hated their udders being touched. More than a few of us got our hands kicked.

But here we were, mid-winter, with the cows dried off and nothing to do. It was the quietest time of all. Don and I would see any companion animals that came in, but today there was nothing.

And then Richard rushed into the office and the calm was shattered. 'Everyone, let's go! Silver Pine Farm has a bloat outbreak.'

With that, all 10 of the vets in the office got up and rushed out to their vehicles.

'Make sure you have a surgical kit and plenty of suture,' Richard told me as I was about to get into my truck.

I'd only read about bloat outbreaks in my textbook. All I could remember was that the rumen could fill up with gas if cattle ate too much high-protein feed too fast. I knew from what I had read that the gas-filled rumen pushed up on the diaphragm, making it hard to breathe. If they were lying down and having trouble breathing, you needed to stab the rumen with a knife to let the gas rush out. Eventually, if the gas was not released, the cattle would suffocate.

The farm was close by. Our fleet of utes tore down the highway and pulled up at the same time. The farmworker was in a panic.

Cattle were sprawled across a paddock of kale. A few

lay swollen and unmoving. Half a dozen were lying down, open-mouth panting. Their rumens were swollen out to preposterous sizes, creating enormous bulges on their left sides. Some of the cattle had been stabbed already by a farmworker, and now stood calmly.

I pulled a bloat knife from the back of my truck and jumped the fence into the paddock behind Richard, who was surprisingly nimble for a man in his late fifties.

He pointed to one of the panting animals as he ran past. 'Stab that one!' He stopped at the next cow.

I vaguely recalled something about measuring two hand spans back from the top of the ribs. I saw Richard stab down and a burst of gas and grass fly up around his face. Seeing where he stabbed the rumen, I decided to copy him. I plunged the short knife down into the cow's swollen abdomen, expecting a burst of gas. Nothing happened. Her tongue was dark purple, sticking out from her mouth as she heaved desperately.

'Pull the knife down and back, towards her knee — make a decent cut!' Richard shouted as he relieved another cow.

The other vets had fanned out across the paddock and bursts of gas were ringing out. It sounded like a group of campers letting down air mattresses. I pulled the knife down and back towards her udder and the gas blasted out, sending stomach contents into my face. The smell of gas and grass was so intense I almost gagged. The cow gave a great sigh and took some deep breaths.

Richard shot past me to help another vet, flashing me an amused grin behind his mask of green splatter. I must have looked the same. The stabbed cows began to settle, their crisis temporarily over.

Together with the other vets and the farmworker we herded the non-critical bloated cows into the yards. We ran them up into the race one by one, and put a stomach tube down their throats and into the rumen to relieve the gas, then pumped in bloat oil. The protein-rich kale had formed a reaction in the rumen that had caused a foam to form, blocking the expulsion of gas. The oil would break down the foam and resolve the problem.

I felt sorry for the young farmworker as he pumped the oil up the tube from the bucket. He looked only about 19. This was a farmer's worst nightmare.

'They broke through the fence,' he explained as he worked the pump, his expression grim.

Usually, the cows were filled up with fibrous feed such as hay, then exposed to a small section of kale so that they didn't gorge themselves and bloat. These cows had gotten greedy and pushed through the electric wire to have a feast. Sadly, for some of them it would be their last meal. Later in the winter they might have got away with it, as their rumens would have adjusted to the new feed, but this early on it was a disaster.

Richard left two vets to drench the other cows. The rest of us herded the cows that we had bloat-stabbed up onto the rotary milking platform, leaving every second stall empty so a vet could stand beside each cow and stitch her up.

There were 13 cows to stitch, and we all got to work. Working through the relatively small stab-hole to stitch the rumen was difficult and Richard came around to help the young vets. I couldn't see how the cow would survive. Grass had blown out and was stuck in the lacerated muscle layers and on the outer surface of the rumen: these were areas that were usually sterile, separated from the digestive contents. Grass and fluid had fallen into the lower abdomen. It was a mess.

Richard insisted that most of them would live, so we carried on stitching. I flushed penicillin into the area before closing the muscle layers, and then again before closing the skin layer. By the time I had finished, one of the senior vets had finished stitching their second cow. I couldn't believe how fast they worked. The cows were given a long course of antibiotics and pain relief. After that, all we could do was wait and see.

Two weeks later, Silver Pine Farm called the office and told us that two of the 13 cows died. I was sad that they hadn't all survived, but equally surprised that the majority had. I thought most of them wouldn't make it with all that rumen contents inside their guts, but it was as Richard said: cows are tough. I wondered whether there was something to be learned from cows. Maybe every animal has a lesson hidden within, if only we take the time to look.

Later that week I would be needing the resilience of a cattle beast. My life was about to change.

CHAPTER THIRTEEN

DR TARZAN

UP UNTIL THAT DAY I had been thinking of my life as a pot of soup. On the kitchen bench lay a colourful array of ingredients. These were people, experiences, events . . . the positive ones were fresh, tasty morsels that I would throw into the boiling soup, the bad were rotten things that I threw in the rubbish. So far it had been working nicely and I had a fine soup bubbling away.

It was the seventh week into my first job as a vet. I had passed all my exams with good grades. I'd even passed the North American Veterinary Licensing Examination (NAVLE), which would allow me to practise in North America. Amber and I had spent the summer visiting beaches, hiking in the mountains and staying up into the small hours enjoying each other's company. I could still remember her sweetness and soft touch. The pain that followed her departure to Thailand had almost faded as we adjusted to our video-calling relationship. Besides, I would be heading over there to meet her in a month's time.

So what was the problem?

I had no contingency plan. What happens if the soup is knocked from the stove? What if it crashes to the floor, explodes onto the walls, and half-cooked potatoes skid steaming across the tiles?

By the time I got back from the bloat call, it was late on a Friday afternoon. I waved goodbye to my workmates, excited about the weekend ahead. My friends pulled up outside the clinic in a station wagon, in high spirits, too. We were headed to the lake for a stag do.

When we arrived at the serene mountain lake, we were delighted to find a rope swing dangling high from a tree beside the lake. It hung invitingly above the edge of the water on an open gravelly beach. Behind the beach, thick native bush extended up to the foot of the surrounding mountains, skirting them in deep green.

We attached one of our water-skiing ropes to the bottom of the swing. Next, we assigned a group of guys to run and pull it back, to get the swing nice and high before it swung back out over the water.

A few of my mates had a go and soared impossibly high, whooping with delight. I was eager to have a turn. Ignoring a warning stab of anxiety in my gut, I proceeded to the launching point for the rope. Only later would I count all of the reasons why I shouldn't have ignored my instincts. For starters, I hadn't noticed that by then three or four more of the group had joined the pulling team, swelling the group up to about eight. I was also lighter than the last few punters who had been on the swing.

But at the time I did not process this, I just felt an

instinctive uneasiness, which I put down to adrenaline. So I silenced my doubts and climbed onto the rope.

They pulled and I raced backwards, and then up, and up, and up . . . 15 feet . . . then 20 . . . then 25—

CRACK.

The old, weathered rope snapped.

I spun in the air, free-falling, turning to see where I was headed to land. What I saw filled me with horror. Flying in a great arc, I was on track to smack straight into the group of guys 8 metres below me, who were now looking up at my approach in shock. I had time as I fell to process the ghastly scenario ahead. Too much time. How could I *still* be falling? I was going to be paralysed; no — worse — I was going to die. I was falling not into the water, but onto stony ground.

The ground rushed up at me, and I hit with a terrible thud. Every bone in my body jolted and rattled, and I felt a horrific pop in my back as my spine snapped. I lay still, unable to move.

Intense pain filled my whole body, most of it radiating from my back and pelvis. My vision narrowed, and my breathing became shallow and rapid. I fought to stay conscious, but pain pushed me into a deep nothingness. Part of me wanted to embrace the darkness, but another part of me was instinctively fighting against it, not sure whether I would ever wake again if I succumbed to the oblivion.

All the while, my skin was blanching white, my lips turning blue. The muscles in my back were twitching rapidly, and, although I was shivering, I felt hot.

One of my friends had knelt by my head and was talking to me. I didn't hear what he was saying. All I could think about was fighting to stay awake, and how irritating the sandflies were that were landing on my body and arms, biting me. The ground I lay on was not the beach, it was hard-packed stony earth — I'd flown so far that I'd missed the sand entirely.

'Touch my toes,' I croaked. Just speaking was agonising.

Someone reached across to touch my toes, and relief flooded through me as I felt their fingers gently squeeze. I wriggled them tentatively. Thank God, I'm not paralysed. But the *pain*. People were placing jackets over me, but I felt hot and wanted them off. I could hear someone phoning for a helicopter behind me. *Pain*.

A memory of telling Amber I wouldn't do anything stupid just before I left niggled at me. This pang of guilt was interrupted by a wailing siren coming from the nearby township. The shrill sound rippled across the lake and echoed off the surrounding mountains.

Impossibly, the waves of agony began to intensify, each one driving me deeper into an internal hell.

It wasn't long before medics came running across a swing-bridge to the beach. An older woman took charge and rallied my stunned companions. Carefully, they tried to roll me onto my back. Knifing pain twisted through my body, and I cried out in agony. But the woman's stern, determined look was enough to keep them tipping me slowly over until I was lying flat. I gasped and my vision blurred.

To my horror, a different pain began to hit me, even

worse than before. It was my feet. It was as if every nerve in them had been told to scream at me with the intensity of a thousand wasps. The realisation hit me: they must be smashed, too. What part of me wasn't broken?

The medic put a catheter in my arm and started giving me morphine. The pain didn't seem to relent much, but my mind took a half-step back as I entered a dreamlike state. My friends became dark silhouettes against the sky.

A helicopter chattered. Wind and sand blasted me as more medics crouched down, sliding a backboard under me. I stared numbly at the sky as they carried me to the helicopter.

Whatever happened next was a blur of pain, doctors, beeping machines and raised voices.

'Why an MRI?' '. . . doesn't need that to fly . . .' 'My shift should have finished at three . . .'

A friend's hands were holding me down on the bed because my body was involuntarily moving and rolling as if it was trying to writhe itself free of the pain, putting my spine at risk. My buddy's brow creased with worry and concentration as he tried to restrain me without hurting me more. Apparently, the morphine was losing the fight.

Then they were moving me again, this time for X-rays. Both my heels were badly smashed, my pelvis was broken, as was my tailbone and my back.

As fragments of these diagnoses penetrated my consciousness, realisation dawned. Life as I knew it was over. Would I ever work again? Or play sports? Run, or even walk?

New doctors appeared. They had flown to the small coastal hospital from Christchurch. They seemed angry about something . . . 'His pain levels . . .' 'What were you thinking?' . . . 'Give him ketamine . . .'

They injected me, and I began to levitate from my bed until my face pressed against the ceiling. 'I'm in the ceiling. I'm flying away!' I shouted down to them.

Is this what it feels like to die? The world faded.

Amber got a message early that morning, her time:

> Marcus has had an accident, a bad fall. They've airlifted him to the hospital. We are awaiting X-rays, will update you when I can.

She didn't go into work that day, or the next, but sat by her phone in Thailand waiting to find out what had happened.

I didn't have the strength to open my eyes. I could hear beeping and muffled voices. Something was in my throat, the endotracheal tube. I wanted to pull it out. Instead, I reached up and tapped on it to try to tell the nurse to take it out. It felt like an eternity before she finally did, and I groggily opened my eyes.

I was in a different room, surrounded by medical equipment and monitors. My family was sitting on chairs backed against the wall. When my mother saw that I was awake she came over to my bedside and explained that I had been flown up from the West Coast to Christchurch during the night. My family had been waiting for me at Christchurch hospital, and had watched as the medics had wheeled me unconscious from the ambulance into the intensive care unit.

My throat was raw, and I could manage only a few words.

'Call Amber . . . Tell her . . .' I paused, hesitating. The sound that croaked from my lips sounded like someone else's voice. The voice of a sick old gaffer, not a young man.

'Say I'm okay,' I concluded.

My dad frowned, clearly disagreeing with my assessment, but he called her anyway.

The drugs had sapped every drip of adrenaline and endorphin from my body. I felt awful. When Amber picked up the call, I could hear her soft, scared voice on the other line punctuating my dad's flat-voiced narrative. He didn't tell her I was okay. He told her the truth. I didn't dare try to speak and have my rattling voice breathe emphasis on his words.

A few days later I was moved from ICU to the trauma unit, where staff bustled about the six patients in the room. I awaited a visit from the junior registrar on his daily rounds. In my experience, when faced with their first patients junior doctors can generally be divided into two groups:

those in the first group will be visibly nervous and shaky, stammering, their sentences punctuated by glances at their notes. They are — rather appropriately, I might add — unsure of their clinical decisions and conclusions. This group of doctors will likely ask for help from a senior, even if it may feel embarrassing to admit their lack of certainty.

Then there's the second group. These are the types who revel in a pompous false confidence, so deeply invested in the façade that they have even begun to fool themselves. They charge ahead, spittle flying as they regally pronounce the diagnoses, some even miraculously doing so before the tests have been run. Just like I did, with Tiger's rotten tooth.

As the doctor on rounds swept through my hospital door that afternoon, I could only pray that back in the day I hadn't exuded the same blazing overconfidence.

His lab coat was spotless. If I wasn't mistaken, he'd ironed it that very morning. His blonde hair was meticulously styled. Matching its shade was a thick, bristly moustache. I can't tell you why the thing annoyed me, but annoy me it did.

His eyebrows pinched together as he frowned at his clipboard. 'Oh dear. Hmmm, yes, not good at all,' he tutted, his head shaking slowly. 'Broken L1, bilateral calcaneal fractures . . .'

He looked up suddenly. 'Right! Unfortunately, you have the most painful possible orthopaedic injury. *And* not one, but *two* counts of it.' He paused for a beat, then charged on. 'The heels are filled with nerves and are extremely sensitive. You're in for a terrible time.'

'Oh,' I responded flatly. 'Well, I appreciate the honesty, I guess.'

But if I thought he was finished, I was mistaken.

'If somebody was my arch-nemesis and I wanted to hurt them very badly, and let's say . . .' he paused, deep in thought, 'let's say I was only allowed to break two of their bones. Well, I would get a hammer and smash both of their heels.' He pointed at my thickly bandaged legs. 'Those are the worst bones to break. By *far*.'

'I'm glad I'm not your enemy,' I winced, growing uneasy. This guy had clearly missed the med school module on soothing bedside manners. 'So will I be able to run again?'

'Run?' he chortled. 'You'll be lucky if you can walk normally.'

I felt my heart sink as I let the assessment wash over me. 'Can I go back to work, as a vet?' I asked nervously.

He glanced down at my patient notes. 'Farm vet? No way,' he declared. 'In the clinic with the cats and dogs, *maybe*.' With that, he gathered his notes and strode from the room.

I felt as if I had been left holding a torn balloon, sitting silently in the dark, the merry memory of the party hovering ghost-like beyond my grasping hands. Not a farm vet anymore? Never run again? Changing my career already?

These questions floated in my head for the next few

days, until a tall man in his sixties walked into my room.

He spoke quietly with a nurse, who nodded and left. Turning, he crossed the room to my bed. He wore a buttoned-collar shirt and dress pants, and his eyes were kind.

'Hi, I'm Matthew, your surgeon. I'm going to fix your feet,' he said warmly.

'Fix them? But I was told they were a virtual write-off and I wouldn't be able to work as a vet again.'

He smiled reassuringly. 'A vet? I have a guy who had the same injuries as you who is now back in his unit in the military. You'll be able to work again.'

'Run?' I pressed, hope surging through me.

'Yes, run, jump, swim. It might be uncomfortable, but you'll be back.' His expression was mild, but it darkened as he continued. 'Now, I must warn you, this is the most painful orthopaedic surgery that I do. I usually do one foot, and then a few weeks later the other, because the pain is so bad.'

'Do them both.'

Matthew regarded me for a moment, weighing up something. 'Are you sure? You will have some very bad nights.'

'Yes, do them both as soon as you can.' I wanted to get out of this place.

Matthew hadn't been exaggerating. After the six-hour surgery, I spent the next few weeks in unimaginable pain.

Sleep abandoned me, and my nights were reduced to glaring at the hospital clock, willing its hands to move faster. Metal screws had been driven through the bone fragments that were my heels, and were now holding them together, along with metal plates and an artificial bone graft. It was agony.

Four excruciatingly long weeks later they released me from hospital. After two months recovering at home, my wheelchair had become an extension of me. Balancing on the back wheels was as effortless as standing had once been, and the muscles in my arms had bulked up from the constant workout.

Don was looking at me, his concern plain.

'Are you sure?' he asked for the third time.

'Don, they said three months. It *has been* three months,' I pointed out.

'But shouldn't there be a physio or someone with you?' he insisted. Despite his words, I detected his resignation and edged my way to the front of the chair.

'Last week I ventured into the wide world of two-legged folk, daring to visit a fancy restaurant. I spotted my friends' table on the far side of the place. This awkward beast,' I gestured to my wheelchair, 'didn't have a hope of navigating the labyrinth of tables and chairs that lay ahead. Half the bloody restaurant stood up to move tables and chairs. I'm not sure what was worse: the pitying glances of the compassionate, or the tight-lipped scowls of the irritated. So pass me the crutches,' I ordered. 'I'm done with this bloody chair.'

He frowned, hesitated, then handed the crutches over. I heard his sharp intake of breath as I began to lean forward onto the crutches, my weight shifting to my arms. Then I pushed. My feeble thin legs did little, but with the strength of my arms I was able to haul myself to my feet. I wobbled, and Don seized me by the arm. I shot him a look, and he stepped back reluctantly.

I let the crutches fall to the ground and threw my arms into the air.

'I'm enormous!' I declared.

'Take it easy,' Don cautioned.

'Don, I'm leaving the world of thighs and belts, boots and buttocks behind me!' I sang happily. Don continued to watch me nervously, but then smiled despite himself.

I couldn't believe how *tall* I was. Had I grown?

Then the pain began to stab at me. The fat pads that cushioned the bottom of my feet had wasted away, and the resulting sensation was comparable to standing directly on the heel bones. Despite their screams of complaint, I wasn't willing to part with the moment, though.

My thoughts were interrupted by a knock on the door. Don and I exchanged a questioning look. We weren't expecting anyone. Don moved to the door and swung it open.

My heart stopped. It was impossible.

It was *Amber*!

My mouth opened; my mind went blank. Then she was walking towards me and laying her hands gently on my shoulders, her soft brown eyes holding mine. Her skin was impossibly smooth, the tone as warm as a rich olive. My mouth opened and shut uselessly as I tried to think of something to say. She couldn't be here; she should be in Thailand.

She saved me by stepping forward and gripping me tightly. Her warmth shattered the ice from around my heart. I felt her compassion, her sweetness, like a warm breeze. Don had tactfully tottered off by the time I found my voice.

'You're here?' I asked stupidly.

'I'm here,' she said.

CHAPTER FOURTEEN

TWIST & POP

MY BOOTS CRUNCHED ON GRAVEL as I stepped from the warmth of my truck into crisp winter air. It still amazed me to walk upright on my own two legs again. The morning sun streaked the fields gold and illuminated the fog from my breath. Had there been a breeze, the cold would have bitten, but the cloudless morning was still. The air smelled of freshly cut grass and cattle.

Amber's visit had been short, but sweet nonetheless. My feet were still painful, but I found that if I gritted my teeth and was efficient with my jobs I could press on.

A familiar pang of nerves accompanied me on what was one of my first farm visits after my accident. When you're called to a cow having trouble calving, you truly never know what you're going to find when you arrive. She could be lying down in the mud, exhausted from the effort. She could be wild and aggressive due to ketosis. She could be near to good facilities, or she could be in the middle of a back paddock. The calf might be dead or alive. It could be in any number of positions: head turned back, one or two legs back, upside down, coming backwards. It could be a mutated calf with multiple legs or heads, inside-out, full of fluid; it could be twins, the mother's uterus could be twisted . . . the list goes on and on. So, naturally, you can drive yourself nearly mad — as I had done more than once — trying to anticipate what lay ahead.

I secured my calving gown behind my neck and pulled on my long plastic gloves as I approached the cattle yards. Regardless of what lay in store for me, there was one certainty: it would be messy. I spotted a tall Friesian cow waiting silently, her head held in the metal head bail. Her journey from the paddock had left the black-and-white hair on her underbelly flecked with mud. Her tail, arched out behind her, flicked nervously as she shifted her weight uncomfortably.

A flustered man came out of the dairy shed, wiping his hands on his overalls. His hair was speckled with silver and his face wore the lines of a man who spent all day in the sun.

'Morning,' the farm manager greeted me. Then he frowned as he followed my gaze to the cow. 'Yeah, she's a problem, all right. Real tight. It's like when I put my hand in, it can't get through to where the calf is.' He mimed his attempt to reach the calf. I'd heard this line before and knew what lay ahead.

Be wary of pattern recognition. I could almost hear the professor's voice and see his wagging finger. Easy for you to say, I rebutted his spectacled shade.

In an ideal world of lab tests, X-rays and MRI, clinicians

can summarise their findings, write their possible diagnoses and begin to rule each one out as they work down a diagnostic pathway. On a farm, it is just you and your instinct as you stand before the silent, cud-chewing mystery that is a sick cow. A whiff of sweet breath, a shifting of weight, a grunt, a look in the eye, air bubbles in the poo, or a key phrase from a farmer is the most you can hope for, so the practitioner has to pounce on every clue they can. I told the farm manager I'd take a look, and he promised to send some help over while he finished off a few jobs around the farm.

I made my way over to the cow. After cleaning her back end, I filled my hands with lube and rubbed it over my arms. I extended my fingers, bunching them into a cone, then put my arm in, reaching down into her uterus. As my hand moved towards her cervix, it twisted down and to the left: her uterus was twisted anticlockwise. A twist can happen if a cow moves the wrong way, or if a calf thrashes in utero, making it impossible for the calf to pass through the cervix during birth.

As I was reaching this conclusion, I heard the distinct sound of gumboots thwacking against the backs of hairy calf muscles, and glanced over my shoulder to see two fresh-faced farmhands approaching. Gangly twins who looked around 18 years old were making their way over to witness the unfolding drama.

'What's 'appnin' 'ere thinn?' one asked.

'Irishmen?' I asked.

They nodded happily.

'We jus' arrived, actually. Came to take a look — see how ye run things down 'ere, with yer big herds an' all. So far, it's been good crack.' He turned to his brother, who nodded in enthusiastic agreement.

They were new to the New Zealand farming system, where herds are often 10 times the size of those in Ireland.

'It's a twisted uterus,' I said, answering their earlier question. In truth I was relieved to see them, because what we needed to do next would require all the strength we could get.

'Whad's dat thinn?' The second boy's voice rose and fell like a fountain.

'The calf has rolled upside down inside her, twisting her mother's uterus. We need to roll the cow to correct it.'

The Irish lads glanced at each other excitedly.

I began to wrap the big cow with a long rope as the Irishmen watched, creating a series of loops that would tighten when pulled. One around her neck (that would not tighten), one just behind her front legs and one just in front of her udder and back legs. I left 2 metres of rope extending out behind her.

I turned to them. 'Are you ready, fellas?'

They exchanged another look. 'Reddy fur what now?'

'I'm going to open the gate here, and she's going to walk out into the pen. Keep hold of that rope there behind her and follow her out. I'll join you on the end of the rope, and, when I say pull, pull like there's a couple of Englishmen at the other end.'

They beamed at that.

I opened the gate, and she strolled out with the Irishmen, quite literally, in tow. Once she was walking in the pen, I ran to join them with the rope.

'Pull!' I yelled.

We pulled. The rope tightened around her chest and stomach, she staggered to the left, then to the right. Her knees folded, and 600 kilograms of cow crumpled down to the ground. I ran to her and held her head down before she could think about standing back up. I looked back at the Irishmen, who were panting and grinning from ear-to-ear.

'We're not done yet, lads — we still have to roll her. We're going to roll her anticlockwise,' I told them.

This was so she would 'catch up' to her internal anticlockwise twist. The key was to put weight down on her abdomen to hold the uterus in place as we rolled her. The process was often a chaotic scramble of swearing men and flailing hooves. It wasn't unheard of for farmers or vets to get kicked or crushed in the process. I would need to be careful.

The cow looked at me calmly. I had to admit, so far she had been obliging.

'Good lady. We'll have you fixed soon,' I assured her.

I spotted the manager scurrying between tasks and called him over. Now we were four. She'd fallen with her left side on the ground, which was a good start. I assigned one Irishman to the front legs, and the other, along with the farm manager, to the back legs. Some vets lean a long plank of wood on the cow's abdomen and a keen volunteer 'surfs' on it while she rolls. This is to keep the uterus in place while the cow rotates. As much as I enjoy an early morning cow-surf, there wasn't a plank handy, so I knelt on her belly instead. I placed my knees on her abdomen just in front of her thighs, then I checked that my helpers were in position. They nodded to me in turn, and I readied myself.

'GO!' The men grunted and heaved, and the cow started to roll under me. Feeling like I was running on a barrel, I walked my knees backwards to keep from flipping over with the cow. Then, with one final grunt, the cow rolled over completely. I scrambled off her and hurried around to check if it had worked.

I put my hand back in. Damn. She was still twisted.

I looked up at the panting group. Rolling the huge animal had taken its toll.

'Sorry. One more time, fellas.'

They nodded without complaint.

We repeated the exercise and heaved her over a second time. Again, I put my arm in, silently praying it had worked. I found the cervix open. The twist was gone.

'It's open,' I announced happily.

The Irishmen's smiles widened, and the farm manager nodded his thanks before hurrying back to his long list of chores.

But as I felt the approaching calf, I realised my job was far from done. The calf had its leg tucked back, tangled in the foetal membranes, making it difficult to free. Ten minutes later I was starting to feel the burn in my arms and wondering if this leg would ever come up. The Irish pair had found a perch on a nearby rail and chatted idly as I worked.

Finally, I was able to get my hand cupped over the hoof to protect the cow from its sharp edge, and then gently flick the foot and leg forward. The calf was now presenting correctly, front feet first. I pumped more lube in, gripped both of its front feet, and pulled. The calf came out easily, but it was surprisingly small and showed no signs of life.

I glanced up at the Irish boys and shook my head; they nodded, understanding.

I put my arm back in, and to my surprise a tight membrane pushed against my hand. Panic flooded me; her uterus must have ripped when she rolled, and now her bladder was poking through. Then, piercing the fog of my panic, from the back of my mind came a small, rational voice, telling me that this was a twin coming, still in its sac. Desperately, I pushed against the membrane, but to my dismay I couldn't feel a calf inside.

'All right?' one of the Irishmen enquired. My face must have betrayed me.

I nodded and told them they could carry on with their morning. What I needed was time. If it was a twin, it would be pushed up by the cow's contractions so that I could feel it. If it was the bladder, it wouldn't move. And if it truly was her bladder, she was done for.

I returned to my truck and called Don. Maybe he would know. Maybe he could reassure me that it was just a twin on its way. He was at a call-out of his own on a farm nearby; if needed, he could come and help.

With Don on the line, I pinched the phone to my ear with my shoulder and put my hand inside her once more. The tight fluid-filled membrane was sitting in the pelvic canal. I ran my hands over it and described it to Don. Then I pushed, hoping that this time I would meet the reassuring feeling of a twin's foot, or maybe a head. The structure *exploded.* A torrent of fluid poured out of the cow's backside, drenching me.

'What?! What is it?' Don shrieked, his panicked tone matching mine.

'The fluid. It . . . it smells like urine!' I wailed.

'What? OH MY GOD! I'm coming right now!' Don yelled into the phone.

But when I put my hand back inside the cow, I felt a calf's hard, pointed hoof.

'No . . . no, stop . . .' I chuckled, warming with relief.

'You can feel a foot, can't you?' said Don, joining my laughter.

The membrane was just the birth sac, and the fluid was normal birthing fluid.

I could picture his smirk as he drove. He was already assembling his tale for the senior vets.

'Don, listen now: you will NEVER tell the other vets about this. NEVER. Swear it!' To my surprise, between his gasps of laughter, he gave his word.

I put my hand back into the cow and felt the twin's head, which was turned to face its own backside. It wasn't going to be able to come out like that. I hooked my hand over its nose and pulled its head up towards me. For a second time that morning, I pulled on a pair of spindly legs. This time, the calf came out alive. I folded at the waist as I caught the heavy creature and lowered it to the ground.

She lay there a moment, then lifted her head and shook away the birth fluids. She seemed happy to be experiencing the world on the right axis. So was I.

Later that day I had a realisation. Every time a farmer called me for help with a calving, he had already tried getting the calf out. The birth sac was always broken. On top of this, twins were rare, and often they were born without help due to their smaller size. Well, I knew now, and I vowed that it would be the last hysterical call I made to a colleague, screaming that an animal's organ had exploded.

My only consolation came from the tentative conversations I had with my classmates in the weeks to come. As it turned out, I was not alone. The rural vet's first spring is trial by fire, filled with victories, heartbreaks and even disaster, some too woeful to record. The work is physically, mentally and, at times, emotionally exhausting. When that spring ended, I decided it was time to move on and leave New Zealand.

The season wasn't the only thing coming to an end.

Amber had called to tell me that our relationship was over. The break-up was more painful than my bone-shattering injury. I felt shaken, wounded and vulnerable. As the call ended, I pulled my truck over, unable to see the road through the tears. She wanted consistency and stability. I craved spontaneity and adventure. She wanted Canada. I longed to feel the sun and dive the sea.

CHAPTER FIFTEEN

MAUNA LOA

A SPRAY OF COOL, SALTY WATER hit my face. The waves boomed as they hit the rocks below, but I didn't dare look down. I was clinging to a cliff face, halfway down. Going back up would be just as hard as continuing on down. This was the sixth time my life had come into real danger since I'd stepped off that first flight to Indonesia.

The first time had been when roadside robbers had wielded sharpened machetes against me. Next, a rogue wave had sucked me into its thick lip, before smashing down on the reef, splintering my board. I missed a terrorist attack by two days, endured a relentless hold-down by a wave that could have passed for a small hill in the Philippines, and finally a tiger shark paid me a fleeting visit, perhaps welcoming me to the warm waters that he called home here in Hawai'i.

Hawai'i's Big Island is a giant active volcano, filled with excitement and danger. This, combined with the fact that it sits right in the middle of the Pacific Ocean, catching powerful swells from all sides, makes it an adventurers' paradise. That was why I had come and now here I was, clinging tight to a crumbling cliff on a moody, humid night. Had I taken the time to reflect more deeply, I may have seen my relentless flirtation with danger as a way of coping with pain, both physical and emotional. But, perhaps fittingly, the life joyride I'd embarked upon left no time for reflection, no space for the very thing that might just bump a man back to the realm of order.

The first drops of rain began to fall as the moon vanished behind thick clouds; now the only light came from the hotel restaurant perched on a cliff nearby. I looked up at Ryan, who was peering at me from the cliff edge. Since leaving the special forces, he'd discovered a new way to get his adrenaline fix: taking visitors to the island on daring — verging on insane — homespun missions.

'Are you sure you've done this before?' I shouted up to Ryan, my voice strained with nerves.

He gave me a thumbs-up as splashes of rain dripped from his nose.

'You're almost there! I'll throw the bodyboard down to you once you're at the bottom!' he shouted, pitching his voice over the thundering waves.

I looked over to the balcony of the nearby restaurant, which in turn looked across at the section of cliff we were descending. A crowd had gathered, excited by the prospect of seeing a bunch of hooligans fall from a cliff, be eaten by tiger sharks, or both. The patrons had been alerted to the fact that something unusual was going on when they had seen our troop scurrying through the hotel holding snorkelling gear and bodyboards.

A huge floodlight directed from the hotel restaurant onto the ocean below attracted krill, which in turn attracted enormous manta rays. That was what we were here for. I could see them now, gliding below the surface like great shimmering carpets under the swell. These colossal rays can grow up to 9 metres in wingspan. I took a breath and continued my downward climb.

My mask and snorkel flapped against my chest as I negotiated the cliff's jagged, slippery handholds. Finally, my feet touched the wet rocks at the bottom. I let out a breath just as a dark wall of water surged straight for me. In moments I'd be smashed into the cliff behind and then dragged back across the sharp rocks. The spectators fumbled their phones from their pockets to capture the impending catastrophe.

'Catch!'

I looked up to see a bodyboard cartwheeling through the air. I snatched it from the sky and leapt at the oncoming wave with a split second to spare. My board just cleared the top of it, and I skimmed over the black torrent rushing below me. As the wave made its booming collision with the cliff, I paddled away from the rocks. My heart raced. Adrenaline surged. The growing crowd cheered and clapped from their viewing platform.

The next member of the group had already begun their descent under Ryan's guidance. They were blessed with a lull in the waves and made it safely to the water.

The sea looked ethereal, shimmering and dancing under the light. Maybe our launch had scared the great manta rays away. I prayed I hadn't just risked my neck for nothing. Minutes passed and the diners began to trickle back to their meals. I shivered and hugged my shoulders as I floated in the darkness.

Ryan called out and pointed excitedly. A manta ray was heading straight for me. I lay still as the great black shadow materialised beneath me. She was massive. I scrambled to put my mask on, then dipped my face in the water. She took up almost my entire field of vision as she glided past, a great diamond of grey. Her back was dark, with two small areas of lighter grey behind her mouth.

It was at this point that I remembered that the Australian naturalist Steve Irwin had died while swimming with rays: when one startled, it had sent its razored barb into his chest. But that was a sting ray, I hurriedly reassured myself; manta rays don't sting.

This manta ray peered up at me curiously before drifting on. I watched as she slowly moved her wings up and down, flying effortlessly through the water. She banked into a lazy turn, then faded into the darkness.

I lifted my head out of the water and looked up at Ryan, who was sitting with his legs dangling off the cliff, unphased by the rain. He gave me another enthusiastic thumbs-up. Then he pointed ahead of me, so I lowered my mask once more and dipped beneath the surface.

This manta swam below me, then started to pitch up, beginning a great loop up and back towards me. I watched in amazement as the vast creature inverted, now swimming upside down directly towards me. His huge mouth gaped, filtering krill from the water. In a few seconds, I was going to be sucked right into a living cave. The great hollow mouth was just a few feet away. I was frozen, my limbs heavy.

Then the manta began to pitch back down, dipping just inches below my face. I lowered my arms slightly, and let my fingers run along the underside of his belly as he passed. The skin was rough and leathery. He continued his loop back down to the sandy bottom and glided away.

Still unsure whether what I had just seen was real, I paddled towards Ryan, who had now descended the cliff and was hanging from a hold a few feet from the bottom.

'They're really something, huh?' he said.

I nodded.

'How do we get back up?' I called.

'Yeah, well, this is the hard part!' he shouted back.

'The *hard* part? What was climbing down then?' I demanded.

'The fun part!' he laughed easily.

His voice was lost in the boom of a wave crashing against the cliff. The spray showered down on the turbulent water in front of me.

His words rose over the waves once more. 'Ride a wave onto the rocks and beach yourself; I'll grab you and pull you up!'

I looked at the rocks, shadowed in the low light. Even in the darkness, I could make out the razor-sharp barnacles.

'Ride a wave onto *those*?' I objected, outraged. 'This is a kamikaze mission.'

He just grinned and pointed, showing me where I needed to beach myself.

I waited anxiously for the swell to come. The first wave surged up the rocks, then sucked back out, draining off the sharp edges to expose my cheese-grater landing pad.

A second wave came and went.

'You need to take the next one!' Ryan urged.

I paddled closer and felt a surge behind me, pushing me forward. I paddled hard with it and was launched onto the rocks. Ryan reached down and caught me behind my upper arm, pulling me up onto my feet.

'Hold on!' he urged. I crouched low as the water sucked back, trying to pull me with it. I grabbed a rock with my left hand, and Ryan held onto my right arm with an iron grip. The water cascaded past me, and we held firm. The bodyboard dangled from the leash on my wrist.

'Now climb! Quickly!' he barked. I scrambled up the cliff as the next surge approached. A plume of water exploded around me as I climbed higher, just out of the ocean's reach.

'Landed first time, not bad,' Ryan mused as I climbed past him, headed for the cliff top. I threw my board up to some of the wiser group members who had elected to watch from land.

'What happens if you fail the landing?' I asked, once my feet were firmly on safe ground.

'Cuts and scrapes. Sometimes stitches, but so far so good today.'

I joined the others at the top to watch as my snorkel buddy took his turn. He clenched his jaw and rode a huge surge up onto the rocks. Ryan grabbed him, but the swimmer lost his footing as he tried to stand in the rushing water. He toppled onto the rocks and the water sucked him down. Ryan wasn't going to let the ocean have him so easily, though. He clung to the panicking boy's arm as he dangled like a rag doll from the rocks, water falling around him.

After what felt like an eternity, the ocean finished its cascading suck, and he was able to see the rocks and grab a hold. As he scrambled towards Ryan, a second ocean surge rushed in. There was no way he would get up the cliff in time. The water scooped him up and launched him forward, dumping him back down on the sharp rocks. Ryan had been forced to let go to avoid being pulled in himself.

Seconds later it drained back, rolling the boy across the rocks. He would have almost certainly fallen, dripping with blood, into the notoriously shark-infested water but for his desperate snatch for the rocks. His fingers closed around a knobbly hold, and he dangled, muscles straining. The water churned.

Ryan took no chances; the fellow wouldn't survive a third hit. In the time it takes to draw a single breath, he was down and pulling the battered boy up. Minutes later the pair crested the cliff to join us. The boy folded over, panting. His chest and stomach looked as though a clowder of cats had used him as a climbing tree. He was shaken, but didn't appear to have any other injuries. The seawater had mixed with blood to form a diluted red webbing trickling down his shins. Ryan glanced down at the bleeding knee.

'Just the one scratch! That's a new record,' he announced proudly.

Three weeks later I clasped hands with Ryan in a warm farewell and made my way inside the airport. My time on the Big Island had been punctuated with thrills and danger. Before I'd departed that volcanic playground, I had witnessed the rescue of a tourist with a broken neck, a father swimming in powerful surf, his infant child perched happily on his shoulder, and raced a flash-flood through dark, winding lava tubes. The tunnels were so long and perfectly round that they could have as easily been formed by giant worms, chewing their way through the volcano. I smiled as I remembered sliding down a steep section of tunnel, the water rising around our feet.

Deep inside, a faint voice that held some affiliation with the idea of consequences tried to speak. I think it had always been trying to speak to me, but I'd just grown adept at ignoring it. Today, it broke through.

I wondered if this was what people felt when they jittered on the edge of a high-diving board, or perhaps decided to watch rather than leap onto a perilous rope swing. I shivered at that last memory.

Mortality wasn't something most 25-year-olds think about. Then again, perhaps that frayed rope was what had put the fire under my feet and sent me on this reckless sprint at life. The near brush with death had made me realise just how finite my life was. Before that day, I had assumed I would have a long life and die in my bed as a 90-year-old. Now, I had a new sense of motivation to do the things I dreamed of doing sooner rather than later. After all, we never know when our time is up.

I had been wanting to travel the world since I was 18, but I had kept saying 'after my degree', 'after I've worked a few years', 'after—'

'Your *bag,* sir,' the airport staff member snapped, breaking my reverie.

'Oh, yeah, sorry,' I mumbled, swinging the heavy pack from my back onto the baggage conveyor belt. I should have felt happier considering I was checking into a flight to Maui, but my mood had darkened after saying goodbye to my new friends on the Big Island. I was growing tired of making friends only to lose them a few weeks later.

I let out a great heave of air and reached for the boarding pass in the clerk's hand but at the last second she tilted her wrist up and I grabbed thin air. My surprised expression must have been amusing, because she smiled at me for the first time.

'You're a surfer?' she asked.

'Yeah,' I said, my brow furrowing.

'Talk to a local before just paddling out at whichever spot you've read about on your favourite blogger's site, or whatever it is you kids read,' she told me.

I looked at her for the first time. Her deeply tanned skin had the lines and spots of a woman who had spent her life in the sun and ocean.

Anticipating my question, she went on, 'I'm tired of seeing tourists drowned, eaten or beat up.'

'Eaten?' I blurted, taken aback.

'There've been fifteen shark attacks in the past twelve months where you're headed.' With that, she handed over my boarding pass and looked over my shoulder to invite the next unfortunate passenger to the desk.

CHAPTER SIXTEEN

MAUI

I WALKED OUT of Maui's Kahului Airport into tropical sunshine. The passenger pick-up area was deserted. Before I'd left for Maui, my mum had told me she had a cousin on the island named Rena. 'She'll be there to pick you up, but just a heads-up, she's a little . . . wild,' her message had read.

I glanced down the empty road and began to wonder whether Rena had been one of the unfortunate 15 eaten by sharks. The few other passengers from my flight were long gone. I waited another half hour, and had just decided to call a taxi when a black SUV towing a Zodiac boat sped around the corner. It lurched to a stop, and a woman in her fifties popped her head out the window and grinned.

'Chuck your stuff in the back. We're going boating! Huh-haaa!'

I returned her smile and threw my pack into the tray. As I made my way to the front seat, I spotted a box of beer and two packs of sushi sitting on the back seat.

'Say hi to the kids,' she said as I climbed in, thumbing back to the goodies. 'They don't complain much. We'll enjoy them on the water, yeah?'

Suddenly it was clear which part of the family my wild streak came from.

'Let's do it,' I agreed, feeling at home already.

I'd been on the island for only an hour, and I was already skimming across the waves. The beers and sushi were secured in a dry bag, beside which lay my snorkel and fins. The sun sparkled, shimmering gold on the turquoise water as the island shrank behind us. The wind whipped my hair, and schools of flying fish leapt and glided just feet away, matching our speed. There was a smaller island far across the channel from us.

'That's Lanai,' Rena said, pitching her voice over the growling motor. 'Have you heard about the tiger sharks?'

'A lovely lady at the airport was kind enough to warn me,' I called back.

Rena throttled back so she could speak over the motor; its roar hushed to a low grumble. 'One of my friends was on duty with the lifeboat when he saw a Swedish tourist out in the water. Well, what was left of her. She'd been caught in a feeding frenzy. She was just a head and shoulders. Keep an eye out for fins! Huh-haaa!' She whooped again.

A few minutes later I drew Rena's attention to a disturbance in the water. What I was seeing defied reason. A long, silvery fish was ploughing along the surface of the water, only it was moving sideways. Its momentum pushed a hill of water ahead of it, and behind it was a grey nose. Before I could gape any longer the thing had vanished, leaving only a strange sense of confusion and curiosity behind.

'Rena,' I asked, 'was that a shark chomping on a fish?'

'Looked like it,' she answered easily.

I swallowed and peered into the water, wondering what else swam below.

'Hey!' she shouted, pointing across the water ahead of us. 'Look at that!'

I looked over just in time to see an enormous humpback whale launch up from the water. He hung in the air, seemingly suspended in time, before coming down with a great crash. The resulting splash looked like a bomb had gone off. A second later the loud clap of his impact slapped my ears. I gaped in shock.

'Yeeeeeehhhhaaaa!' Rena whooped.

'That's *insane*,' I breathed, awestruck.

'You think that's something? Look there.' She pointed to our left. I could just make out two black-coloured backs cresting the water, tipped with small, curved fins. Rena cut the engine and we floated in sudden silence.

'They're heading straight at us,' I pointed out, excitedly. We were about to be run over by humpback whales. I pulled my fins on and slipped my mask over my eyes and nose. Rena watched me cheerfully, unconcerned.

'You go in, but I might have to move,' she warned me. 'Sometimes the bull whales get a little, well, bullish. I'll come back and pick you up if I do.'

For a moment that inner voice concerned with consequences tried to pipe up, as thoughts of the Swedish tourist's messy end combined with thoughts of the bottomless ocean below me hosting those prehistoric hunters, ancient and hungry. I firmly silenced it. After all, this was a once in a lifetime moment.

I tipped back off the boat, holding the mask against my face. Small bubbles filled my vision as I righted myself. The sound of water slapping against the boat and the soft breeze above vanished. I kicked slowly, descending, feeling the resistance of the fins against my feet. I pinched my nose, blew, and was rewarded with the high-pitched squeak of air squeezing past my eardrums. The pressure behind them eased. I dived further and equalised again.

Once I'd reached around 7 metres, I waited, looking through the deep blue in the direction from which the whales had been approaching. The visibility astonished me; I could see at least 70 metres through the water.

Two immense black shapes were materialising in the distance. As they approached, I could see their enormous tails moving up and down, the slow motion propelling them with surprising speed. Long, graceful flippers extended horizontally from their barnacle-studded bodies, guiding their movement through the sea. As they got closer, I could make out every detail: battle scars along their sides and white underbellies, the black fist-sized bumps that mottled their faces, and eyes, dark and intelligent, regarding me with curiosity as they drew near.

The mating pair drew level with me. Only at this point — when they were mere metres away — could I appreciate their almost-impossible magnitude.

The world slowed and then stopped in the exchange. The tiger sharks were forgotten. Even my need for oxygen was gone, as I floated, captivated. Then, as quickly as they had approached, they moved away, their tails waving goodbye.

I reluctantly kicked back up to the surface, slowly letting my breath out as I did. The bubbles danced up with me, little stemless mushrooms that shimmered as they rose to the surface. Rena smiled down at me from the boat.

'That was beyond incredible,' I declared.

Rena pointed down at the water for a second time. 'Looks like Hawai'i is really turning it on for your arrival, little bro,' she said.

I put my face back down into the water to see what she was pointing at. To my astonishment, a pod of dolphins had appeared and were swimming nearby.

I spun back up to face her. 'Dolphins now!' I exclaimed.

I put my face back into the water and watched the dolphins whirl around one another. They circled the boat a few times before continuing their fishing expedition. Reluctantly, I hauled myself back onto the Zodiac, water pouring off me onto the deck. Rena seemed to sense my inability to speak, and wordlessly chugged us forward.

Minutes later, a back the size of a tanker truck breached the surface just 20 metres away from our boat. This whale was headed right at us, but, unlike the earlier pair, this one was moving with determined speed. I reached for my mask.

'Not so fast,' Rena warned. She had her hand on the throttle and was watching, alert.

Then I understood. The big bull had remained on the surface, and was accelerating.

'Shoots!' Rena cried, as the bull thrashed its tail down and sped at us. Whooping, she sped the little boat away just before the massive creature collided with us. I could have sworn she held off the evasive manoeuvre as a final ploy to make me soil my boardshorts.

Hooting and cheering, she turned us back towards Maui and opened the throttle. The boat's nose lifted, and half a dozen empty beer bottles clanked back to join her as she sat easily at the back of the boat, holding the engine's throttle arm. I grabbed the rope trailing from the bow and turned my face from the spray as we punched through choppy water.

I clutched the memory of the whales, hugging it close to me, pulling it in. This lifestyle, as glorious as it was, was only temporary. One can only wander for so long before our deeply ingrained need to be part of a community draws us back.

I was to return once more to the complexities of cases and surgeries, claws and fur, grateful smiles and tears of mourning. My job hunt had already begun. I was moving to Canada.

CHAPTER SEVENTEEN

A SUMMER FREEZE

MY WEEKS IN MAUI had been breathtaking. It was a stroke of luck that had landed me there in March, during the humpback whales' mating season. But now I had to leave because I had run out of money. I had just exited a video call with three elderly Canadian men who seemed less than impressed by my stunning backdrop — a sprawling palm on a restaurant balcony. My tanned face, unruly hair and mention of surfing through Asia for the past five months only sharpened their scowls. From a dim office in British Columbia, they deemed my gallivanting to be inappropriate for a professional, and decided that the sliver of skill gleaned from my meagre two years of practice had likely been doused by the sea.

I looked at the next clinic on the list. Arctic Animal Hospital, St John's, Newfoundland. I pulled up a map. I regarded the small island off the east coast of Canada, not too far from Greenland, then shrugged and dialled the number.

The young man seated next to me on the plane glanced up, perplexed. Alfred had a sharp nose, a pointy chin and blonde hair cropped into a bowl cut; his pale skin looked as though it had never seen the sun. He'd just told me he was on his way home to see his wife and young child. Like most of the other men on the plane, he was returning from an oil run in Alberta, cashed up.

'Yer dowin' wat baiy?' Alfred asked, puzzled. 'Yer tellin' me you cudn' fine anover playse to do yer vet work?'

I took a long time to answer, partly because he was hard to understand, partly because I didn't have a decent answer. His frank disbelief at my city of choice stirred a mild panic. What exactly was I doing heading to this remote place, and why did everyone sound half Irish?

Finally, I found my voice and began to muster a defence. 'Uh, well yes, there were lots of vet jobs around actually. Vancouver Island, BC, Alberta—'

'And ye bloody well come 'ere!' the jubilant chap laughed, slapping his knees. 'Oh, good Lord!' Tears appeared in his eyes as he struggled for air. Eventually, he pulled himself together, only to lose it again.

Passengers began to crane their necks to see the source of the commotion.

'Do ye know how you're gettin' te town from thee airporr then, baiy?' He raised his eyebrows, an amused smirk playing at the corner of his mouth.

'The bus?' I ventured. This appeared to be the funniest

thing I had said all afternoon. Alfred exploded.

'Bus? BUS?' Alfred, noticing he had gained an audience, looked around the plane to bring the other passengers in on the apparent absurdity of my suggestion.

Some of the passengers began to chuckle.

'There's no bus,' Alfred managed between gasps, shaking his head in disbelief. He finally took a few long, calming breaths and spoke again, forcing composure. 'Look . . . me dad will give ye a ride.'

The plane dropped below the cloud line, and I peered out the window. The island was vast, scattered with dark patches of pine and rugged rock formations. Cliffs lined the coast, wild waves crashing below, and the ground was covered in snow. It was summer.

'Snow?' I exclaimed, disbelief in my voice.

'Yes, baiy. *Snow*,' my new friend replied frankly. His cheeks had flushed red from his laughing fit. 'Ye know,' he began, changing the subject, 'I went tih thee vet once.' Alfred flicked his wrist and limply injected the air in front of him, then held out his hand to me, his eyebrows raised. 'Hundred bucks.'

After a long drive, we pulled up to my hostel. 'Good luck, baiy. You'll need it with that little pair of shorts on! Ha!' Alfred called as his dad joined the laughter.

I grabbed my bag from the back of the ute and waved goodbye. My feet squeaked in the dry snow as I tentatively made my way to the hostel down the sidewalk of an ancient-looking street lined with brightly painted two-storey houses.

Once inside, I signed in at the desk and a young German man with white-blonde hair took the paperwork and handed me a key.

'So, why are you here?' he enquired politely.

'I honestly don't know,' I told him.

He laughed. 'Sounds like you'll fit in. There's only a handful of travellers here; you'll get to know us. We're headed to the pub in an hour — you're welcome to come along.'

A few hours later I stepped into a bustling pub with my new companions. Our boyish faces and lack of sea-weathered beards distinguished us from the others in the room. In one corner a young woman was singing movingly about a boy who yearned to leave the island, but couldn't bring himself to leave his mother behind, all alone.

I was lost in the music when a hand slapped down on my shoulder. I turned to see a familiar face. It looked like Alfred from the plane, only his eyes were looking in different directions.

'Alfred?' I queried.

The musician's melody rose above the noise, singing of the mother's weariness and the young boy's burden.

'Yer—' He leaned back and almost fell, before grabbing my arm and righting himself. 'Yer a good . . . a good lad.' He patted my cheek, smiling. 'A good lad.'

The singer began a new verse; the boy's father was lost at sea. Alfred followed my eyes to the singer.

'Beautiful, isn't it?' he slurred. 'The song's called "Sonny's Dream". Might be she sings of your alter ego, my lad. For every boy on an adventure, there's one stuck at home.' He smiled an odd smile, a smile that didn't reach his eyes. 'First it was the sea, then the wars, now . . . oil.' Sadness held him as he watched her sing. He seemed to sober up for a moment. 'A land of lonely daughters, mothers and wives missing their men . . .'

He sighed, and, as suddenly as it had appeared, his melancholy was gone. He reached forward, took a freshly poured beer from the bar and pushed it into my hand. His eyes drifted apart once more, and he raised his glass. 'Welcome to Newfoundland!'

The streets of St John's were impossibly steep and narrow. Some intersections had roads coming from five or six different directions and angles. Some streets hid behind buildings, others were undetectable given the angle at which they came up to meet the intersection with a bigger road. I looked all five ways and then pedalled my new bike across the bumpy street.

As I rode, my mind drifted to thoughts of Amber. I couldn't help but wonder if she knew I had moved to Canada. I daydreamed of her knocking on my door to tell me that it had all been a foolish mistake. She still loved me, she'd say, before falling into my arms again.

I shook my head, exasperated at my stupid, stubborn heart, and turned down a steep road. I picked up speed; the icy air whipping at my ears. My hands stung, and my teeth chattered. I'd taken a bike against all advice because I had no choice. With my budget, it was that or an old car falling apart from the rust caused by Newfoundland's salted winter roads.

I accelerated down the hill, approaching the next spider-webbed intersection. Passing the waiting row of cars, I pulled my rear brake and—

My front wheel locked. My seat launched, and I flew over my handlebars. The steep street gave me the extra flying time I needed to get my legs under me, and I landed in a flailing sprint, floundering into the middle of the intersection, cars skidding to avoid me. Still, I remained upright as I reeled to a stop. My bike finished its own cartwheel and rattled down onto the concrete beside me.

The busy road stilled. Onlookers stared at me as I stood there, bemused by my lack of injury.

A lady popped her head out of her car window. 'You all right?'

This seemed to slap me back into my body. I nodded, collected my bike, and trotted away from the attention. I had just discovered that the front and back brakes on bikes are reversed in North America.

My hair was wet when I reached the clinic on the city outskirts, and my hands had darkened to an even deeper shade of purple. One of the nurses greeted me at the door.

'Aye there, lad!' Her welcoming expression changed to one of surprise as she took in my shivering form. 'What are ye at, baiy? Yer looks like a drowned rat. That's no good now, get inside.' She ushered me in and handed me a towel.

Once I was semi-dry, she walked me to a large closet, from which she pulled a white coat off a hanger. The name Dr Taylor was embroidered on it.

'You already sorted me a coat? Thanks,' I said.

She nodded grimly. 'This belonged to one of our vets; he was the best kind. He passed away last year.'

'I'm sorry.' I put the coat on solemnly.

'You're the only man here. There're twenty women.' She watched me, weighing my reaction.

'Great,' I said, my face a careful mask.

She laughed. 'Ha! You've no idea, Marcus. But don't worry, baiy. Ye've got me. I'm Kate.' She reached out and gripped my hand. 'And by the way, I likes girls. I'm not a man, mind, but at least we can talk about ladies together, eh?' She jabbed me with her elbow companionably.

An hour later I was in the consulting chair. My first patient, a chocolate Labrador puppy, sat on the table in front of me. He slid down onto his belly, resting his chin on the consult room table. He was woebegone and somewhat subdued, the result of an excited snatch at a seemingly harmless piece of squid.

The fisherman who had brought him in was tall and lean, with a scruffy goatee, weathered skin and short, dark hair.

He spoke up in a booming voice, filling me in on the back story. 'Oh roigh', ah tell ye, baiy, 'ee jus champ down on thee 'ook there, I never had toime to grab 'em.'

I couldn't understand him. He was from 'round the bay', which I'd quickly learnt meant he was from one of the small seaside villages out of town. Out there, they spoke their own dialect. Luckily, I could see the fish-hook hanging from the puppy's lower lip, so the issue was strikingly obvious.

'All right, not a problem. We'll take care of it,' I said.

'Yes, baiy. But 'eey now' — he looked around before leaning in, lowering his voice to continue in a stage whisper past the back of his hand — 'keep the cost lowish, would ye?' He winked at me.

'I'll do my best,' I offered.

He handed me the puppy, and I took him into the back room to show Kate. The hook was inside the puppy's mouth, sticking into his lower lip, the barbed end buried deep into the pink tissue.

'Oh! It's a sin! I hates these,' she complained. 'Draw up a light sedation dose, and get the pliers,' she asked one of the assistants. Kate then turned to me. 'You're doing this — I'll talk you through it.'

Disentangling and pulling a fish-hook from a dog's

mouth was a scenario that had never even crossed my mind.

Minutes later, Kate laid the drowsy puppy down on his side, holding him in case he moved despite his sedation. I injected local anaesthetic into his cheek, then looked up at Kate.

'You need to push it all the way through, then cut the barb off. If you just try to pull it out, it rips the tissue and makes a real mess,' she told me. 'You also need to be quick about it.'

I carefully pinched the puppy's lower lip with my thumb and index finger, rolling it back to expose the hook. The puppy let out a sad, sleepy whine. The hook looked deep enough that there wouldn't be far to go before the barb would be visible.

I gripped the hook with a pair of needle drivers. We usually used them to hold a needle while suturing a wound, but they worked perfectly for this. I winced as I thrust the hook the rest of the way through the puppy's lip and the barb surfaced from his skin. Kate passed me the pliers. I snipped the barb from the end of the hook. Once it was cut, I carefully rotated the hook and removed it from his lip. I held it up to Kate.

'The furry fish is free,' I announced.

'Speaking of fish,' she said, a cunning look on her face. 'It's time we get you initiated . . .'

CHAPTER EIGHTEEN

THE INITIATE

'STAY WHERE YE AT till I comes tah where yer to!' we shouted, echoing the bearded man at the front. It was a class, of a sort. I was learning to speak 'Newfie'.

'Aie. Nat bad,' he grunted, leaning back. 'That's a command meaning "Stay there, till I arrive".'

'Bring out the fish!' he bellowed over his shoulder, keeping his eyes on us. The kitchen doors opened, and a portly man came out holding a huge dead fish.

'Who's first then?' he asked. The room fell silent.

Finally, a woman walked forward and kissed the fish, right on its cold, dead lips. The patrons roared their approval. The man handed her a shot glass filled with a dark liquid, and a hush fell once more.

'It's called "screech",' he said, sensing her confusion. 'It's our favourite drink, see. Strong and good for warming the belly on the cold seas!'

She eyed the mysterious concoction, then tipped the glass back, wincing as the contents went down.

Then the massive fish was pointed in my direction.

Blank eyes advanced towards my face. The kiss was cold but, to be fair on the fish, I'd had worse. Cheering rang out and a shot glass was put in my hand.

I felt a tap on my shoulder. Kate from the clinic. I turned to see the other nurses watching me, a mixture of pity and amusement.

Kate held up her phone. 'We have to go, you're on call, remember?'

'The other vets said it's usually quiet on weeknights,' I complained.

She shrugged, ushering me from the warmth of the pub into the chilly night air.

Kate and I arrived at the clinic to find a car waiting in the parking lot. We opened the clinic, hurriedly prepared a few things, and then let in a middle-aged man and a boy who looked around 12 years old. The dark-haired boy held a cat swaddled in a blanket, his slender arms carefully cradling the package. The cat was struggling to breathe.

At my request, he gently laid the cat on the examination table. She lay limp, breathing hard. There was blood matted in her dark-grey fur. The boy sobbed; his hand pressed to his face.

'Trix ran across the highway and was hit. Adam saw the whole thing,' the man told me, patting his son on the back.

Adam's sobs grew louder. I looked at the cat's face. Her eyes were half closed. Then, with a great effort, she lifted her head at the sound of Adam's grief, and I saw. Her *jaw.* Her jaw hung from her face, barely attached. Severely fractured jaw, possible cracked ribs, ruptured diaphragm likely, multiple fractures. Trix's life was fading.

'Get oxygen, and an IV line ready, please,' I said to Kate.

She hurried away.

'I'm so sorry this has happened,' I began gently. 'I have to be honest: this doesn't look good.'

I laid out the options, and a cost estimate, and then I described the surgery that would be needed to repair the jaw if she lived through the night. After a few moments of thought, the father made a choice, a choice that many unfortunate pet owners are faced with at the most unpredictable of times. When he had sat down for dinner an hour earlier, the last thing on this man's mind had been coming here to make this kind of decision.

Often it's very hard to know what to do. As an owner, you can spend thousands of dollars trying to keep a dying animal alive, hoping that they may pull through. In the process, you may end up extending their suffering to no avail. But sometimes, even when things look hopeless, by some miracle of fate, after the treatment, they make it. You get to live on with your beloved family member, fresh gratitude for them in your heart. The alternative to attempting treatment is making the call, there and then, to have your pet put down — a decision made even more difficult when your child is in the room.

As the vet, all I can do in these moments is set out the facts as clearly as possible, an estimated chance of survival given treatment, and some comfort. I'm frequently asked, 'What would you do if you were me?' Some vets avoid answering such a question, understandably not wanting to make decisions for their clients. I choose to tell them honestly what I would do if I were in their shoes. Every little bit helps with the most difficult of decisions.

'I think we should put her down,' the man managed, his voice thick with sadness.

His son burst into fresh tears. He grabbed hold of his father's shirt tightly, looking up at him.

'Trix! No, Dad — *please*!' the boy wept. 'Can't we save her? *Please*, Dad.' Tears ran down his face and dripped onto the floor.

The poor man looked at me helplessly. I knelt beside the boy. He wouldn't meet my eyes.

'Adam,' I said gently, 'I understand that you love Trix a lot. But she's badly hurt, she's in a lot of pain and she's dying. If I try to save her, she might stay alive a few hours longer, but she will likely still pass away and will suffer during that time. I know you love her, and that you don't want her to hurt.'

Adam turned and pressed his face into his dad's shirt.

'We can give her some medicine now and she won't feel any more pain. She will go to sleep peacefully, then her heart will stop.' I watched the boy as he mulled over my words. 'I think your dad is making a good choice. It's a difficult decision, but it's the kindest thing to do,' I told him honestly.

Adam turned his head slightly and peered at me with

one watery eye. Then his face disappeared once more into the makeshift haven that was his dad's shirt.

I looked up at his father, who nodded solemnly.

Kate was already returning to the room with a tray of needles, syringes, swabs and medication. She had intuitively included the pentobarbital, the medication we use to put animals down, in the kit. I shook my head at her, and she gave a short nod to show she understood. She began to draw up the medication while I did the paperwork with the father.

'Would you like to say goodbye to Trix?' I asked the boy.

He nodded and walked up to her, gently patting the top of her head. 'Bye, Trix,' he whispered. 'You were the best cat.' Pain crumpled the father's face. His eyes began to water along with his son's as I explained what to expect during the procedure. An overdose of anaesthetic . . . her heart will stop . . . there may be muscle contractions . . . Unfortunately, I knew the lines too well.

'Are you okay for me to go ahead?' I asked, containing my own emotions so that I could continue to operate.

He nodded, now holding Adam, who had turned around to watch.

The boy had stopped crying and looked on, red-cheeked, as his life-long friend's breathing slowed, then stopped. Her absence of life left a stillness, a finality, in the room. We silently packed up, wrapping Trix back in her blanket.

The door shut behind them as they left, leaving a sudden silence. During the day the clinic bustled with life, but at night it felt eerie.

Kate's phone rang. We looked at each other for a moment, surprised.

'Again?' I wondered aloud. I wanted nothing more than to go home and take some time to digest the events of the evening.

Kate answered her phone. I watched her carefully, trying in vain to read her reaction to the barely audible babbling.

'His *what* is cut?' she asked, squinting. 'His throat?!' she exclaimed, shooting a stricken look at me. 'Bring him down right now.' She hung up.

I must have looked as horrified as I felt, because she changed her tone quickly.

'It will be okay. We can just do what we can do, the rest is out of our control,' she reassured me.

Together, Kate and I laid out all the things we thought we would need on the bench in the treatment room. Stitch kit . . . bandages . . . butorphanol . . .

The door burst open, and a young couple walked a golden retriever into the room. They were holding a blood-soaked bandage against his throat. At least he was still on his feet.

'When did it happen?' I asked quickly.

'Twenty minutes ago,' the man told me. 'I think he ran into the corner of the coffee table or something . . . I'm not sure.' He shook his head.

I sat the dog down on the floor in the corner and got

to work. I asked the woman to straddle the dog and hold his head still. I pulled their rough bandage off and hastily pressed a swab against the bleeding cut.

'His name is Bilbo,' the man continued as he knelt beside me to watch.

Thankfully, the laceration had just missed the jugular, otherwise Bilbo would not have even made it as far as the clinic.

I asked Kate to give him some butorphanol for pain relief, and began to clip away the fur around the swab. The woman was doing a good job of holding his head still for me, and Bilbo was surprisingly cooperative.

After about five minutes of pressure, I lifted the swab to confirm that the bleeding had stopped. I put some sterile lube into the wound, and then gently clipped the last of the hair away. Now I needed to inject local anaesthetic and then stitch the wound closed.

Most dogs needed to be sedated for this, but occasionally they are calm enough to let you operate without it. Bilbo seemed pretty good, and, besides, it was 10 p.m. and I was about ready for bed. Kate slipped a muzzle over his jaws, then I injected the local anaesthetic. He whined a little, but otherwise let me go to work.

I had only begun pulling the edges of the wound together with the first stitch when Kate's phone rang again. I swallowed my disbelief and concentrated on my task.

It was a dog having a seizure. I heard Kate ask them to put a blanket under its head and then bring it down as soon as they could. She hung up and crouched back down to help.

Then her phone rang *again*. We looked at each other anxiously.

'Busy night,' Bilbo's owner said.

The newest caller told Kate that their beagle was lying on the floor panting rapidly, unable to move. Kate asked them to bring it down right away. I began to give up any hope of sleep.

By the time I had finished the last stitch and cleaned Bilbo's wound, Kate's phone had rung three more times. There were five patients on the way, and the first of them was already pulling up.

Bilbo's owners thanked us, and then the woman graced me with a sympathetic look. 'I hope you don't have work in the morning.'

A weak laugh was the only response I could muster. Of course I did.

It was after 2 a.m. when we finally locked the clinic door. We had been able to treat and send home all of the patients but one. The beagle that had been lying on his owner's floor panting was in heart failure. We had to keep him in the hospital overnight, starting diuretics in an attempt to clear the fluid from around his lungs.

'I think that's a clinic record,' Kate said as she drove me home. 'And on your first night on call. Damn. You've got some special luck.'

My eyes were heavy, and I had the uncomfortable

sickly feeling of being grievously exhausted. My face hit the pillow, but it was a long time before my mind stopped buzzing enough for me to fall asleep. It wasn't until I meditated on my upcoming weekend surf trip that the graceful gift of sleep carried me away.

CHAPTER NINETEEN

BEST KIND

I RUBBED MY EYES and walked out into the living room as the morning light streamed through a gap in the curtains. The weekend had finally arrived. A relentless honking was coming from the street. My housemate parted the curtains and peered outside.

'They're here,' she announced in her thick Ghanian accent.

Sika was the one responsible for the impeccable tidiness of the flat, a sharp contrast to the first three I had looked at before hastily pouncing on this one a few weeks after I arrived.

'They're in a white van,' she continued. 'Where I'm from, people who get into vans with random guys don't fare so well.'

'Unfortunately, I think that's a universal rule,' I grunted, slinging my backpack over one shoulder.

It was indeed the surfers. I had spent weeks trying to find someone who knew where to surf on this remote rock. It was surrounded by the ocean, so I figured there had to be a surfing spot *somewhere.* I finally got a lead at a pub — a guy giving me the phone number of a local girl, saying she might know something. She didn't, but gave me another number, and here we were.

'If I don't come back, you know what to do,' I said.

'What? No, I don't,' Sika replied.

I tucked my beaten-up old board under my arm and walked out to what looked like an old delivery van idling ominously on our quiet street. Someone had left the board at the hostel, and I'd bought it from the manager for 40 bucks. He'd told me the previous owner hadn't found any surf and had given up, so disillusioned he'd even left the board behind.

My breath steamed out in front of me as I approached the van. Even though it was early summer, the morning sun lacked any real warmth. I breathed warm air onto my free hand, wondering what I was in for. The back doors swung open, and a thick-bearded man reached out to take my board. The back of the van was empty apart from a small wooden stool, which was plonked in the middle. The large, curly-haired fellow sitting in the driver's seat turned around and noticed me looking at the stool.

'Dats ur seat, baiy!' he pointed. 'It slides around a bit, but it's not too bad.'

'Thanks for having me,' I said, climbing in to take my place on the stool. The doors swung shut with a bang. There weren't any windows in the back, and no surfboards in sight. The driver became a silhouette against the grey sky that shone through the windscreen.

'Easiest kidnapping of my life,' he said.

We looked at each other for a few long seconds. Then his face cracked into a smile. We began to chuckle, me somewhat nervously, then we crescendoed into hoots of laughter.

'Ha! I got you!' he shouted through a toothy grin.

His friend climbed into the passenger seat. 'What's all this, then?' he demanded.

'The Kiwi baiy 'ere thought we were going to kidnap him.'

'Are we not, then?' his companion asked.

'He wouldn't sell for much anyway — he's too skinny,' the driver said as he pulled out onto the road. 'Don't they know how to deep fry stuff where you're from, baiy? I hope you've got a decent wetsuit.' He looked back at me again with an evaluating glance. 'You lack essential blubber!' As he took his hands off the wheel and grabbed his belly, his friend casually leaned over and took the wheel, plainly used to stepping in.

After hours of bumps and a few tumbles from the stool, we were finally paddling out over slow, silky waves. My hands stung as they plunged into the frigid water to pull me forward. I was at last 100 per cent sure I wasn't destined for chains and a grim basement.

The pair had collected their surfboards from a beach house, and had donned thick wetsuits, hoods, gloves and booties. My wetsuit was only 4 millimetres thick, suitable for New Zealand's South Island waters but unlikely to cut it here. These were the same waters in which the *Titanic* had sunk, and I knew how that had ended. Still, it was the best I had, and I wasn't going to pass up a chance to try surfing in remote Canada.

The sun was now setting but was in no hurry to fall, as if the island wasn't ready to let go of the evening light. We were at a remote, stony beach break which only worked as a surf spot every few weeks, when there was a decent onshore swell and no wind. An old, forgotten chapel watched us from the side of the hills that lined the shore.

It felt good to be in the water, even if my feet were already numb. A wave broke ahead of me, and I paddled through it, closing my eyes as freezing spray slapped my face. I gasped as a few icy veins snuck down the neck of my wetsuit. The men were right: I needed blubber. I looked up and blinked.

Icebergs lined the horizon, some of them the size of small islands. I sat up on my board and watched in wonder as the golden light flared off the largest of them, kilometres away. I was trying to decide how big it was when the great mass began to do something strange. My eyes watched what my mind couldn't comprehend. The iceberg began to split in half. The colossal pieces rolled apart like two nations parting ways. My mouth opened in disbelief. Three breaths later I jumped at the thunderous *crack* of fracturing ice.

The waves weren't powerful, but they were glassy and fun. I paddled into the first of a set, letting the surge of water carry me before I popped up onto my feet. The board accelerated down the face of the wave, and I bottom-turned to pull back up towards the lip so I could drop in a second time. I was leaving the white water behind, so I cut back into the breaking wave, then away again before it swallowed me. No matter how far from home I am, the joy of playing in nature always fills me as I ride. I surfed half a dozen more, before I completely lost feeling in my limbs and had to paddle in.

It was 30 minutes in the shower and three cups of tea before I stopped shaking and a hint of feeling returned to my toes. Thankfully, my new friends' house was right beside the surf break. That's why their boards weren't in their van. They served up pan-fried fish and potatoes, laughing when I told them that the last place I had surfed was Hawai'i.

'Only the bold surf here,' the van driver said, putting a steaming plate in front of me. 'Or the nutters,' he added jovially.

I nodded my agreement, biting into a potato.

'Do you know where we are?' he asked, raising an eyebrow.

I shook my head, murmuring my delight at the taste of the butter-fried fish.

'Grand,' he chuckled. 'These spots are best kept secret. Keeps them special.' He turned to his companion. 'See? I told you we didn't need to put a sack over his head!'

The Newfoundland hospitality was humanity at its most beautiful. Before I left its stony shores I would be invited to weddings and concerts, on boat trips and for meals. They still dance with me now, the warm faces and sad songs of a far away, forgotten land.

CHAPTER TWENTY

MIRACLE SAL

WHEN I RETURNED to New Zealand 18 months later, my hair, which had been cropped efficiently short when I'd left, sat thick on my shoulders. The tips were bleached golden from the first months of the journey spent in the Pacific. Unfortunately, the last thing a farmer wanted when he called his local vet was a hair model for Pantene walking up his track.

I pulled off my woolly hat to scratch my head as I drove back to the clinic. Tying my hair up and hiding it under the mud-spattered beanie had been an easy solution. The farm calls for the day had gone smoothly, and I felt the contentment of a good day's work settling in. As I pulled into the clinic, I was relieved to see the parking lot empty: the last two hours covering the companion-animal clinic looked as though they would be relaxed.

I was washing my hands and arms when I heard the phone ring. Thirty seconds later the nurse on duty walked into the washroom to announce that my evening plans were about to drastically change. She had just got off the phone with a shepherd, George, who had been giving his unconscious dog mouth-to-mouth.

Sally was a working dog, the best George had ever owned. She was the only one left in her family, and George had not bred from her yet. She was fast, quick to listen, and loved her work — all valuable qualities in a sheep dog.

After a long day on the farm, George had put the dogs away and left them for 30 minutes to do a job. As darkness fell, he returned to his truck, where he found a horrific sight. Sal was unconscious in the dog box in the back of his ute, lying under the other dogs. He pulled her out to find her lips blue and that she wasn't breathing. George put his lips over her nose and blew in precious oxygen, which he followed with chest compressions in the hope of restarting her heart, a technique he'd learned from years of resuscitating lambs in trouble at birth.

After some minutes, to his relief, Sal took a huge gasp of air and started to breathe again. The next hour would be the most critical of Sal's life.

George drove to the clinic as fast as he dared. He shouldered open the door and put the still-unconscious Sal on the table. My nurse put an oxygen mask on her while I put in an IV line, relieved to see the catheter thread into her collapsed vein. I lifted Sal as the nurse slipped electric heat pads under her, and covered her body with a blanket. When a patient is in shock, often their body temperature and blood pressure fall, and they are low on oxygen. Correcting this was our top priority.

Sal was in a bad way. Every five seconds her legs and

neck would violently stretch out in convulsions, and her pupils would rapidly dilate in unison with the spasms. Her eyes were wide open but were registering nothing. I snatched a stethoscope from the wall and listened to her heartbeat. It was very slow and had a loud, churning murmur. Next, I took her temperature. Holding up the thermometer, I was dismayed to see the direness of her situation: her temperature read 33.3 degrees — about 5 degrees below normal.

'This looks very bad, George,' I said.

He gave a curt nod of acknowledgement.

As we continued the supportive therapy, I injected diazepam, an antispasmodic, into the IV line. It acted swiftly, halting her rhythmic convulsions, and yet her heartbeat remained weak and her temperature didn't rise. We administered fluids as fast as I could run them into her vein, and oxygen flowed into the mask settled around her muzzle. My nurse packed even more heat pads around her. But Sal wasn't responding.

As I worked, George told me how he had found Sal. I suggested she may have eaten something poisonous. She could have ingested parasite drench meant for the sheep, or any number of chemicals, pesticides and poisons found around a large operating sheep station. Whatever it was, she was now having very bad diarrhoea and her body appeared to be shutting down.

After a long time without any improvement in Sal's vital signs, I straightened, then turned to George. He already knew what I was going to say.

'George, we may have to put her down,' I said.

He regarded me for what felt like an age before he spoke. 'Are you one hundred per cent sure that she can't survive this?' The love he had for Sal shone clearly on his determined face.

It was plain that she meant a great deal to him. Watching her lying limply on the table was as painful as seeing any dear friend facing death.

'I'm not,' I replied honestly. 'I'm ninety-five per cent sure she won't pull out of this, but I'm not going to tell you that miracles aren't possible. We would need to transfer her to the after-hours clinic, and there will be a significant financial cost, but she has a chance. A slim one, but a chance.'

I could see George weighing the cost, considering his options. He could spend a lot of money and still lose her, and Sal really did need a miracle to pull out of this. Later, George would tell me that he saw something in those vacant eyes that told him she was still there and fighting.

His expression shifted to one of resolve as he finally replied, 'If there's even a slim chance, I'll do whatever it costs.'

I nodded and turned back to work on Sal with an even greater admiration for the man's grit.

Minutes trickled by and Sal remained the same. Then, at a glacial rate, things began to move. The rapidly running IV fluids began to restore her blood pressure. Her heart sounds improved a little. Her temperature climbed to 34.4 degrees as the heat pads continued to do their work. She was still blind and unresponsive, but things were slowly moving in a direction that gave me a glimmer of hope.

After a conversation with the after-hours vet to warn him of Sal's state, we rushed her out to George's ute on a stretcher. Then George made a second dash, this time to the animal hospital in town, where she could get overnight care.

The clinic was quiet as we wiped down the now-filthy bench, picked up syringes and bandage material, and wheeled the oxygen tank back into place.

Exhausted, I drove home and crawled into bed. I wondered how Sal was doing, if she was still fighting or if she had succumbed to whatever toxins had invaded her system. I said a silent prayer for her and tossed and turned through a long night.

The next morning, I pulled into the parking lot just in time to see George walking into the clinic, stony-faced. He was clutching the paperwork from the after-hours clinic in a meaty hand. Saddened, I concluded that he had come to clear the bill and Sal was now gone. Preparing my condolences, I followed him into the building, then paused. George stood there in his brown fleece and work boots, grinning at me.

'She ate a bit in the night and even stood for a moment!' he said. 'Shall I go get her?'

'She's here?' I asked dumbly, following him back out to the ute.

Sal was lying on the back seat, unconscious but settled.

He helped me carry her limp frame through the clinic doors for a second time. She was still blind, but her temperature had returned to normal. I tickled the hair in her ear, and she flicked it in response.

George turned to me. 'Look, I don't want to get false hope here. If you think she's not coming back from this, just say so . . .'

I finished my examination, then lifted my head to face George. 'If there was hope last night, there's even more today, George.' It was my turn to start believing.

George agreed that we should keep Sal on fluids and monitor her progress throughout the day. She ate a small amount, but was still unable to stand, walk or see, but there was something special about this dog, I could feel it, too.

The following day, I arrived at the clinic to loud, incessant barking. It sounded like one of the patients was demanding their breakfast in no uncertain terms. A nurse ran to me as I walked through the door to the treatment room.

'Come and see!' she urged.

I moved through to the kennels and peered into Sal's cage. My jaw dropped. Sal was *standing* — and what's more, she was looking directly at my dumbfounded face. Then she barked, a deafening, coarse sound. She was the culprit behind the morning's ruckus. The only other dog in the kennels was the nurse's pug, who raised his head from his nap to shoot Sal an unimpressed glare.

I tested Sal's vision by peeping around the kennel corner at her. Sure enough, she lifted her head to look up at me each time. Sal had made a complete recovery. I sprang to the phone to call George with the news.

That afternoon when he appeared to collect Sal he stared at her, flabbergasted. Sal rushed at him, wagging her tail, pawing his legs, demanding he let her get back to herding sheep.

When I saw George a few weeks later, he told me about his plan to breed from Sal during her next heat. He intended to continue her legacy of fortitude on sheep farms across New Zealand. I have no doubt her pups have grown and are out there now, herding sheep in green paddocks, barking loudly and cheating death, just like their mum.

CHAPTER TWENTY-ONE

AVIAN JAIL BREAK

I SHOULDERED OPEN the back door of the clinic. In my arms was a disorganised jumble of notebooks, food and whatever else I had remembered to scoop up on the way out of the house. I dumped them on my desk and opened the diary on the computer. To my disappointment, I saw a morning schedule filled with nothing but blank white boxes. Nothing?

I wandered out into the reception area, and then cursed as I nearly skidded over, my woolly winter socks sliding on the polished floor. Callie, our receptionist, was holding the phone to her ear, and she looked up at me as a voice babbled in her ear.

'Excuse me for a minute.' She lowered the phone and put her hand over the receiver. 'Ugh. Do we have a tranquilliser rifle?'

I paused as I ambled over to put the jug on, confused. It was not a question I had been expecting. 'We have a pistol, but not a rifle. Why?'

'Something's escaped,' she remarked flatly.

'Something . . . escaped? What exactly has escaped?' I pressed.

Callie lifted the phone back to her ear.

'Hi again. What has escaped?' As she listened to the reply, her eyes began to bulge and her eyebrows lifted. She lowered the phone once again and whispered to me, 'It's an African ostrich. A big one.'

Minutes later I was in the car with my colleague Carl, the tranq pistol in the back and the exotic-animals textbook balanced on my knee. By this time, I had been returning to this clinic in New Zealand as a locum for several years and the staff were used to my coming and going between various expeditions abroad. I often found changes in staff on my return, but not Carl. Carl was a part of the woodwork. With over 40 years of experience, he was a reassuring presence in the front of the truck.

'It says here that they are very difficult to sedate, and are prone to — ugh, wait.'

I lifted the textbook closer to my face. 'Prone to . . . dying. Oh, right. Someone needs to keep the head up and the neck straight at all times, or they . . . die,' I finished lamely.

'Great,' Carl said as he pulled the truck into a long driveway. He flicked down the sun visor as the winter-morning brightness beamed between two tall poplar trees. 'Well, at least it's not running down the str—'

'There!' I pointed at the huge, agitated bird towering above the shrubs.

About 20 metres away a big bearded man stood facing the bird, holding a tall metal gate. The pair appeared to be in some sort of standoff. I noted that the bird hadn't gone far from his pen, and that his pen mate was standing on the other side of the fence, obviously enjoying the morning drama.

'Easy boy. Eeeeeasy boy,' the man soothed. The ostrich arched his neck defiantly, puffing his wings out.

The man spoke to us without taking his eyes off the bird. 'You guys know how dangerous these things are, right?' His voice was tight.

'We know,' I assured him. Ostriches can kick hard enough to kill a lion.

'Right then, grab a gate,' he commanded.

I looked at Carl, and he shrugged, hefting a nearby gate to hold in front of him. I took one, too. It was heavy, 3 metres tall, and tricky to manoeuvre among the shrubs. What's more, I could see I would need to climb up a retaining wall to get to the posturing bird.

We quickly decided that it was better to try to herd the bird back into his pen, using the gates, before risking the option of a tranquilliser. The problem was that the bird's athletic leap over the fence had landed him on the high piece of ground that bordered the farm's driveway.

The first thing we needed to do was push the escapee off the retaining wall to get him back to the pen. I heaved my gate up the retaining wall onto the ground above, and carefully climbed up after it. The towering bird was just metres away, eyeing me with suspicion. He ruffled his black-and-white feathers, irritated.

'They're not good at pushing,' the man told me. 'Brace yourself against the gate and he will just bounce off it if he goes at you.'

I noticed the man was standing a good deal further back than I was as he hollered his instructions. I was trying not to breathe too hard as I advanced towards the bird. I watched him through the metal grating of my improvised shield as the distance between us closed. The ostrich turned towards me and lifted a leg to reveal long, dark talons. One swipe with that leg would tear me open. I couldn't help noting how alien the creature looked, with his bald head and enormous eyes atop a long, sinuous neck. The corners of his pink beak curved down, making him look like a disgruntled old man.

Carl and our self-appointed coordinator had climbed up after me, and were forming a shield wall to my left. As I closed the distance between myself and the agitated bird, I crab-walked to my right to try to join my gate with the outside of the ostrich pen's fence. Carl and the owner had formed their shield wall to my left and were moving in the same direction. There were 3 metres left . . . then 2 . . .

Spotting the closing gap between my gate and the pen fence, the bird made a decisive dash. His huge, muscled legs smashed through the scrub, snapping dry sticks. I took two fast sidesteps, my gate raised, then lowered it with a split second to spare, bracing for impact. I tensed. Just before a collision, the bird slid to a stop, inches from the gate. I let out a relieved gasp.

'See? I told ya! They just stop,' the man announced from the far end of our makeshift shield wall.

The ostrich lowered his head, putting a huge green eye level with mine. I peered back at him. He had enormous eyelashes, and was utterly unafraid of me. Then his attention shifted to my pink fingers gripping the gate. I quickly danced my hand away, guessing his plan.

'He won't bite you! They don't even have teeth!' the man yelled.

I'd heard that line before, in the wildlife ward at Massey University. I had been asked to retrieve a mature male harrier hawk from his cage. The resident vet had assured me that hawks don't bite, and so I was best to focus on controlling the talons. With that, I had plodded off on my new assignment.

I'd approached the cage armed with a towel, and knelt to tentatively open the latch. The hawk stood tense in the back corner, eyeing me nervously. I took a breath, and threw the towel over the bird. To my surprise, he didn't thrash around; he just lay still, now covered by the towel.

I carefully wrapped my hands around the bird, and then slowly peeled back the towel to reveal his needle-sharp talons. I got hold of his legs, grasping them with one hand, just above the feet. I kept my index finger between them to stop them from being pressed together too hard in my grip. This isn't going too badly, I'd thought.

'Are you okay in there?' The resident vet's voice echoed from the next room.

'Yup, I got him — no problem!' I called back, sounding more confident than I felt. The resident vet was understandably nervous: the last student had walked out, hawk-first, into one of the nurses. The bird's outstretched talons had landed directly on her breasts. As if this wasn't bad enough, the hawk reflexively closed his feet, latching down. It took them the better part of an hour to get the riled raptor off her chest.

I slowly withdrew the bird from his cage, holding the feet away from me as I did so. I stood up, holding him triumphantly.

He looked at me with a beady eye and I grinned back. 'That wasn't so bad, was it, champ?' I asked him.

He glanced down at my hand. It didn't matter that I had anticipated his next move. I couldn't move my hands now. His curved beak chomped down on my finger as if it were a baby rabbit.

Now the ostrich was looking at my other hand, and I pulled that one away, too, swapping the other hand back.

'I can dance all day, ostrich,' I muttered. Having said that, clearly I would make little progress like this so I resolved to take back some ground. Cautiously, I took a step forward with my gate, shunting him back a step. He ambled backwards, glaring at me in rage. We advanced like that for the next 40 minutes, me moving the gate line forward and the ostrich making various attempts to get around it.

Finally, we were at the top of the retaining wall. The ostrich would need to leap down to get back into his pen.

I looked at Carl. 'Do we just push him off?'

'Yeah, I reckon,' he answered.

We moved the gates forward a final step. I pictured the lanky creature cartwheeling down onto the driveway, breaking something. On the contrary, he made an elegant turn and hopped off the wall, flapping his stumpy wings as he made a graceful landing. He trotted through the gate and back into his pen, his pen mate moving to congratulate him on his escape.

When the pen's gate was secured, I gave the team a triumphant high-five.

Then I watched as the reunited couple strutted around the pen together, preening and making noises to one another. I felt a pang. How far would I have to travel before I met a bird of my own?

CHAPTER TWENTY-TWO

LORD HENRY

MY NEXT CALL WAS TO AN ADDRESS I'd never been to. I wound up the road in the shade of tall trees, trying to find the entrance. As I rounded a corner a slim, bald man in a flannel shirt waved me towards a driveway, then keyed in a security code to open the formidable steel gate. He walked up the track and I drove slowly behind, admiring the perfectly manicured gardens and centuries-old trees. Tucked behind a high bush-line sprawled a very grand villa, looking more like a palace than a typical farmhouse.

The man turned left and led me away from the villa to where my patient, a 200-kilogram kunekune pig, snuffed and rooted about the ground at the edge of his pen. The kunekune were given their name by Māori. And it's an accurate one, too: it translates to 'fat and round'. Asian in origin, and introduced in New Zealand by whalers and traders in the early ninteenth century, their population got as low as 50 pigs in the 1980s, before a breeding programme saved them from extinction.

The pig raised his head and sniffed the air, snorting his curiosity.

'Toby,' the man said, shaking my hand. 'I'm the groundskeeper here. And that's Lord Henry,' he added, pointing to the pig and shifting awkwardly as he told me its name.

'This looks like a special place,' I said. I was curious, but didn't want to sound nosy.

'Oh, yeah, special place for special kinds of people. Last week—' he broke off, scratching his nose thoughtfully. 'Anyway, I'm holding you up. I'll let you get set up.'

My curiosity about who had been at the estate the week before now well and truly piqued, it was with no little disappointment that I let the conversation lapse and got to work. Anyway, I'd need to keep my mind on the job.

I needed to sedate Lord Henry so I could trim his feet and clean an abscess that had formed on the side of his head. His hooves were starting to overgrow, which can cause lameness if left unchecked, and the abscess could continue to enlargen, causing pain and permanent damage to the pig's face if I didn't take care of it. Generalised infections caused by abscesses are uncommon, as animals' immune systems are adept at walling them off from the rest of the body, but it was best to not take any risks and get rid of them promptly.

As I drew up the sedation, I avoided looking over at the pig. Pigs are clever, and always seem to catch on when something strange is happening. Once they get riled up, catching and sedating them is a circus.

'I used to pin pigs behind a gate to inject them, but they scream so loud it blows your ears out,' I said conversationally as I connected a short IV extension between the needle and the syringe.

The syringe contained ketamine, butorphanol and medetomidine, a powerful concoction that had the added benefit of being reversible with a second injection. I was using a long needle to make sure it penetrated the layer of fat and reached the muscle below. If the medication was injected into the fat rather than the muscle, it would take forever to work.

I showed Toby the set-up and explained the plan. 'If you drop him a tiny piece of food, I'll sneak up behind and dose him up before he knows what's happened.'

Without the extension tube, jabbing a moving pig with a needle and syringe can be a disaster. The moving muscle throws the syringe around, making pressing down on the plunger difficult. Using the extension tube would allow me to whack the needle in and then run behind the pig, loading him up with sedation. I'd once watched a vet stick a needle into a pig's behind without the syringe on, hoping to connect it up afterwards and give the injection. The pig ran off with the needle in his bum and we spent the next half hour trying to catch him. I wasn't taking any chances.

I hopped over the fence on the far side of the pen. The big boar gave a low snort, objecting to the intrusion. A second later, as Toby held a piece of apple above the fence in the other corner, he'd forgotten all about me. The pig waddled over to Toby, looking up expectantly. I circled around behind him and nodded at Toby to drop the apple.

As he did, I took three strides and whacked the needle down into Lord Henry's rump, landing it as he munched the fruit. He grunted, but kept munching. It wasn't until the stinging of the drug hit that he lurched backwards, almost bowling me over. He spun and ran. I gave chase, getting the final 5 millilitres into him before he outran me. I whipped the needle out and retreated from the pen.

As Lord Henry grew sleepy and we waited for the sedative to take full effect, I wondered whether Toby would fill the gap by dropping some more details about the place.

'I love how secluded the grounds are, behind all the trees and bush,' I prompted.

'Yeah, that's what the MI6 guys said, too.' Toby looked guilt-stricken as the words left his mouth, but like a schoolboy with a secret he was longing to divulge he went on. 'They were here, taking notes, making sure the perimeter was secure.'

'You're kidding! MI6? Why were they in New Zealand?'

'They wouldn't say, of course.'

Then I remembered an article I'd read a few days earlier. 'The prince and princess are coming this year . . .'

Toby smiled. 'Yes, indeed.'

It had never occurred to me that the royal family would stay in a place like this. I assumed they would be in a fancy hotel. But it made sense; it was private and secure. I looked at my surroundings with a new sense of interest. Would the prince and princess find the gardens beautiful? Or was it just background noise to them after decades of luxury?

Lord Henry seemed to answer my musings by tipping onto his side and beginning to snore. That was my cue to get back to work.

I headed over to the kunekune, my foot-trimming tool, a pair of straight-bladed secateurs, in hand. For pigs' soft hooves I found they worked best. You'd be astonished to learn how many garden tools are adapted into practice for animal medicine: tree-branch loppers or even oscillating saws for cattle horns, modified pump sprayers for putting lube into the back ends of animals during assisted births, electric disc sanders for cattle hooves . . .

I nudged Lord Henry with the toe of my boot. He was fast asleep and I silently prayed he would stay that way. If pigs wake suddenly and get excited, they are a nightmare to sedate again.

I trimmed away the excess hoof on the first foot without issue. It was satisfying, seeing the foot restored to a healthy shape. As I worked on the next foot, Lord Henry let out a low groan and flicked his ear. By the time I got to the last foot, he was pulling it back after each lop of the blades. Clearly, I was running out of time.

Getting the dosage of sedative right for a pig is hard. It's not like there is a set of scales to stand them on, and their compact shape makes estimating their weight a challenge. At this point I could top Lord Henry up with more sedation, which would give me about 20 more minutes to work on him; but it would also make him harder to wake up again, an added risk. Or I could just press on and hope he didn't get up and bolt. For now, I decided to forge on.

I drew up some long-acting pain relief and injected it under the skin. While the ketamine and butorphanol would provide pain relief for a few hours, this would last a few days.

I pulled out a scalpel blade, eyeing the fist-sized swelling on Lord Henry's face. When I touched it, the pig grunted, irritated. The abscess was soft, and lancing it would allow it to drain. I glanced over at Toby, who was looking on, clearly intrigued to see how the hyper-speed operation would play out.

I grasped the blade between my thumb and index finger, making a fist with the blade sticking out the bottom. I eyed the target, then held my breath and slapped my fist down, lancing a hole just below the centre of the angry mound. There was a burst of pus, and Lord Henry's eyes snapped open. I froze, willing him to give in to the soporific drug and go back to sleep. Slowly his eyes closed once more.

I could not afford to pause any longer. I flicked the blade down a few centimetres to make a decent opening, which would allow the abscess to properly drain. This time when his eyes opened, he grunted indignantly. I gave the abscess a firm squeeze, and Lord Henry lurched to his feet, then drunkenly trotted across the pen, leaving a trail of custardy pus in his wake. He plonked down on the far side. After a few huffs he rolled onto his side, snoring once more.

As I picked my way through the mess, I couldn't help but muse at the two worlds coexisting in this rural idyll: one where tuxedo-clad MI6 operatives shook (not stirred) the best dry gin and vermouth, topped out with plump olives, the other in which a latex-gloved vet expertly accumulated the ingredients of the veterinary cocktail — blood, shit, piss, pus and hair.

I returned my attention to the task at hand; if I didn't get a move on while Sir Henry was still woozy, it was more likely to be me, not some cocktail ingredients, that would be shaken once the cantankerous boar awoke from his unexpected siesta.

I decided I could have one more go at the abscess before things became impossible. Filling a large syringe with saline, I crept over to Lord Henry, stuck the nozzle of the syringe into the opening I had made with the scalpel, and blasted, flushing out the wound. This time he almost took out my legs as he groggily staggered to his feet and ambled away.

I turned to Toby. 'I think that's all we can do for today. I'll give him another injection and fully wake him up, so you don't need to worry about him.' Leaving a large animal to sleep out a heavy dose of anaesthetic can be risky, due to things such as airway obstruction, so I prefer to use a reversal drug when I can. Anaesthetised cattle can roll onto their side and bloat, but that isn't a concern for a non-ruminant like a pig.

I caught up to Lord Henry for a final time, and found his

ear vein by putting pressure on the base of the ear, making it rise. Using a small needle I injected the reversal drug, and Lord Henry was awake in seconds, oinking and snorting in confusion.

I asked Toby to call me if the abscess filled up again, or if Lord Henry became lethargic or went off his food. I imagined the Prince and Princess of Wales strolling over to the pen in a few days' time. He'd be sporting polished boots and a waistcoat, an equerry at his side. 'Oh my! Alfred, what on earth is that?'

'It appears to be a trail of pus, my liege . . .'

'Good God!'

Lord Henry returned to happily rooting around the pen, and Toby let his pen mate, who sniffed at the abscess with interest, back in. Lord Henry had had his nails done and his face cleaned, and was all ready for his royal visit.

CHAPTER TWENTY-THREE

FORTUNE

MY BREATH WAS A WHITE WISP as I hosed down and scrubbed my calving apron behind the clinic. I'd just celebrated my twenty-seventh birthday and spring had arrived, the air fresh and crisp. I'd come back from a lambing and, as usual, I was re-running the procedure through my mind as I cleaned.

Mrs Jones had arthritis in her hands and couldn't help the lambing ewes anymore, so she often called me out to assist. With the help of her dog Lucy, that morning I had managed to corner a ewe in the paddock and catch her. Once the ewe was laid on her side, she conceded to letting me help.

The slim black-and-white collie sat and watched as I cleaned the ewe's back end, scooping warm, soapy water out from my bucket. I covered my hands in lube, then put one inside the ewe. I could feel three front legs and two heads in the complicated puzzle.

Like typical siblings, both lambs had rushed to be first, and were now wedged in the birth canal. One of them still had a leg pointing backwards and was slightly behind the other, so after pumping more lube into the sheep, I gently put my hand on that lamb's head and pushed it back. Now free to move, the first lamb came out easily as I pulled it by the legs with one hand, while keeping my other hand cupped over the head to keep it straight.

Mrs Jones smiled as the slimy little lamb lifted its head and shook away the green mucous. I lifted its tiny tail: a girl. Mrs Jones picked her up and put her beside the ewe's head so she could sniff and clean her.

I needed to bring the other lamb's front leg forward before I could get it out, so I reached down past its shoulder and hooked my finger behind its carpus, pulling the leg forward slightly. Then I cupped my hand over the lamb's hoof to protect the uterus from its sharp edges and brought it all the way forward.

It wasn't long before the two sisters were sitting in front of the ewe, blinking the goop from their eyes and taking in the world for the first time.

The clinic door opened, interrupting my thoughts. It was Callie from the front desk.

'Fortune is back,' she announced.

'Don't I have another appointment now?' I asked.

'Well, yeah, but Fortune's owner went to another vet while you were away last week, and she said he looked at Fortune like he was a lamb chop. Anyway, she's happy to wait. She's been here twenty minutes already.'

A little later, I popped Fortune down on the examination table. The wee lamb bleated loudly, his little pink tongue poking out. He held his front right leg up free of the table, bearing no weight on the hoof.

During the early weeks of spring, a consistent influx of sick lambs would be brought into the clinic by lifestyle-block owners. These owners were primarily hobby farmers who worked in the city. Many of their animals were regarded more as pets than livestock, so I treated them as I would any other pet.

'So, Sue, what's going on with Fortune?' I asked the lamb's owner as the tall elderly lady fidgeted beside the table. Of course, I could see the lameness, but I had learned that beginning these discussions with an open-ended question frequently paid dividends.

A few weeks back, Sue had rescued Fortune from her neighbour's paddock in the middle of the night. The newborn lamb had been rejected by his mum, and was dying from exposure as he lay in the rain. He had survived the night under her care, but unfortunately he hadn't drunk any of his mother's colostrum, the first milk a ewe lets down for her lamb. It contains antibodies crucial to a young animal's early development. If a lamb doesn't get colostrum its immune system doesn't develop properly, and it can succumb to any of an array of diseases. Pneumonia, diarrhoea, conjunctivitis and joint infections are some of the common issues.

'The coughing cleared up after the injections you gave

him, but now he won't put any weight on that leg, as you can see there,' she gestured to Fortune.

I took his leg and carefully lifted it at the elbow. I began to feel each joint for heat and swelling, and found that the carpus, which is his wrist, was both swollen and hot. Infected. Sue regarded me from behind her large thick-rimmed spectacles, the concern plain in her eyes.

'Is he going to live?' she pressed.

The million-dollar question.

'The other vet gave him a jab, but the joint isn't improving much,' she told me anxiously.

'He has a chance,' I began, 'but it's not a good sign that he is still having issues after the antibiotics. I must warn you, when they haven't had adequate colostrum, they can relapse, or have other issues come up.'

'Just do what you need to do, and we can see how he goes,' she said, cutting me off.

I could see that she was worried I was going to suggest we put the young lamb down. I looked at the little guy on the table, his wool still short, his floppy tail hanging behind him. He had already had two different types of antibiotics, and I was starting to run low on options. There were others, but I would need to start diving into my toolbox for treating cats and dogs. It was clear that Sue loved this little lamb dearly; he was her pet now, after all.

'I can put him on another treatment course,' I told her, 'but the antibiotic isn't licensed for sheep. I know you don't plan on eating him, but well . . .'

I held up my hands defensively as Sue watched me,

aghast. This part was always awkward.

'I have to tell you, there is a ninety-one-day meat withholding, as it's off-label.' This meant the meat couldn't be eaten within 91 days of giving the medication.

With that conversation now out of the way, Sue went away with seven days' worth of injections for Fortune. I hoped that it was going to be enough for him to get back on his feet.

The practice manager had been surprised when she started to see the types of procedures that some people were happy to have done on the 'livestock' they brought into the clinic. The reality is that the perception of an animal's nature is somewhat flexible. To some people cows or lambs are livestock, to others they're pets. I had done eye removals, cut out tumours, amputated a goat's ear, corrected deformed eyelids, and, in the case of Fortune, I was about to do something I had never tried before . . .

When Fortune came back two weeks later, the infected joint had healed, but because he hadn't been using the leg his tendons had contracted and he couldn't straighten the limb to walk.

Sue looked at me sadly as I tried in vain to straighten his leg.

'This is it, isn't it?' she asked, deflated.

'We do have options left,' I reassured her. 'I can splint that leg and get the tendons to straighten out. It will just take a bit of hard work and physio.'

'Really?' Sue brightened. 'Do whatever you need to!'

I added, 'I must warn you, though. He'll need to come back a few times; it could get expensive.'

'Let's just get him right.'

I would have taken Sue for a rich woman but for the little old car she pulled up in to each visit. She didn't seem to attach a limit to the value of her little lamb's life.

I took Fortune through to the companion-animal treatment room. With the help of a nurse and the companion-animal vet, we fashioned him a splint from the assortment of cat and dog splints we had in a box. Once it was firmly bandaged to his leg, I took him back to Sue.

She put her hand over her mouth as I put Fortune down on the floor. His front leg was now encased in a solid tube, the outer layer a bright-red bandage. Fortune tried to walk to her, dragging his front foot rather than placing it down. I walked over and stood above Fortune, my feet on either side of him.

'Walk down the hall, please, Sue,' I directed.

She walked backwards slowly, and Fortune and I followed her. As he dragged the foot, I picked it up and placed it down for him with each step.

'You're going to have to teach him how to walk with it,' I told her.

I watched her do what I had done as she took Fortune across the parking lot and back to her car. She had a towel down on the passenger seat of the little Toyota, where Fortune sat, as happy as any dog. It was remarkable how little insight a client's car could give you into their spending habits on their animals. You would think someone driving a Range Rover would be the most liberal when paying for diagnostics and treatments, but it didn't always work out that way.

Sue returned a week later with Fortune. I laid him on his side on the table and carefully cut his bandages away, then removed the splint. I picked him up and put him down on the floor.

'The moment of truth,' I announced.

Fortune stood there for a moment, swaying. Then he took a few careful steps. The injured leg was now straight, and he could walk on it.

'Excellent!' Sue gave a little cheer.

'Well, that's it then. Just keep up his milk, and fingers crossed we don't have to see him back here again.'

Sue thanked me as she clipped Fortune's lead back onto his collar and walked him out. A poodle and its frizzy-haired owner watched with curiosity as they passed by.

A week later I was sitting at my desk when Callie from reception appeared again. 'Fortune is back,' she said apologetically. 'His joint has swollen up again.'

I dipped my face into my hands, my elbows resting on the desk.

'I'm sorry . . . I know you've been working hard to get

him right,' she said. 'Sue is in the waiting room.'

I walked out and saw Sue sitting with Fortune in her lap. She looked dejected.

'This is it for Fortune, isn't it?' she remarked glumly as she carried the lamb in her arms to the consult room.

It was the same joint as before, and Fortune clearly couldn't put any weight on it once again. He had an elevated temperature, but otherwise was okay. The concern was that if we couldn't get the joint healed, he would develop chronic arthritis and never be able to use the leg properly. He would suffer, and it wouldn't be fair on him.

Sue looked at me with worried eyes as I pondered his chances of recovery.

'I'll tell you what,' I said, 'let's do three days of the same antibiotic we used for the final treatment, and an anti-inflammatory. If he isn't improving, bring him back on day three.'

Three days later he was back. He'd made no improvement, and Sue was looking at me dolefully once more. Reasonable options were running out, and what was I doing anyway? I had eaten lamb chops the night before, for crying out loud. I was starting to rethink my dietary choices.

'Sue, I'm going to speak plainly to you. Fortune is starting to cost you a lot of money. There are options I can reach for, but we usually only do these kinds of things on cats and dogs. It will be expensive, and it might not work.'

'What is it you're thinking of?' she asked me.

'I would need to sedate Fortune and take an X-ray of the joint. Then I would put a needle into the joint and take a sample to send to the lab. After that, I would flush the joint with saline to try to clear out some of the infection. Next, I would put a tourniquet on his leg and then inject antibiotics into the vein and leave the tourniquet on for about fifteen minutes. It's called a local antibiotic perfusion.'

For once Sue hesitated. 'How likely is that to work?'

'To be completely honest, I don't really know. I have never tried this on a lamb before; I don't think many other vets have either. Often owners are put off by the cost and decide to put the lamb down. I don't hold any judgement towards you, whatever you decide. I don't believe there's any right or wrong answer, just what's right for you. Even by collecting this little guy from the paddock in the storm you've already done so much for him.'

Sue sat down with the lamb, thinking. I left the room to give her some time and drafted up a quote for her.

When I returned, she surprised me by taking a quick glance at the quote and nodding her approval.

The procedure worked. Fortune's joint healed and the swelling reduced to normal. Despite this, Sue was sitting in front of me once again, for what must have been the tenth time. Fortune was now more than twice the size he'd been when we first started treating him.

There had been a complication. He had been using the leg too infrequently during his development, and so the muscles were still very small. He could barely support his weight with it. The leg would constantly give way under him, and he would stumble and fall as he tried to walk. It was a heartbreaking sight.

Sue watched me think as Fortune stumbled once again in the consulting room. By now Sue had compressed 'This is the end of the road, isn't it?' into a single glance.

'You're going to think I'm mad,' I warned, by way of response.

'I already do!' she laughed. 'We're a pair of lunatics. Go on, out with it then.'

'There's hydrotherapy. They only use it for dogs, but I don't see why they wouldn't take a sheep . . .'

Sue cackled. 'You mean swimming with him?'

I nodded. 'Want me to call them?'

'Well, you know what?' she said, an amused sparkle in her eyes. 'At this point, I'm open to pretty much anything. Let's just get him walking.'

The hydrotherapy centre was on a farm run by a kind couple who had converted their work shed into a rehabilitation facility for dogs. They were more than happy to give it a go on a young sheep.

Sue walked the stumbling Fortune in. The couple greeted us warmly and showed us to the pool.

They clipped a dog life jacket onto Fortune while I looked at the long, narrow pool, wondering how they were going to get Fortune in. The man's beard was the same shade as Fortune's wool. He disappeared, and returned pushing a long ramp, which he hooked onto the end of the pool. He then walked Fortune up the ramp, and with a little encouragement got him to step into the shallow part of the pool.

Fortune looked up at Sue with panic in his eyes. It was his first time in water. Sue walked over and gave him a reassuring pat. Then the man walked along the side of the pool, and guided Fortune off the shallow part so that he plunged in and began to 'doggy-paddle' its length. He kept his nose and face pointed up out of the water as he went, swimming surprisingly fast. Sue stood at the end of the pool cheering Fortune on towards her. Once he reached the end, she ran to the other side and repeated her cheerleading routine.

The little sheep got a rest between lengths, and was able to do four or five before he got tired and we called it a day. Sue towelled him off while he shook the water from his ears.

It was almost Christmas before I returned to the pool to see how Fortune was getting on. I was astounded to see him springing across the grass outside the shed. Sue ran ahead of him, encouraging him to chase her. He was no longer limping. His muscles had returned, and he was as fit as any sheep his age.

Sue looked up. 'Look at him go!'

It was Fortune's last day at the pool. Sue walked over

to me and handed me a box neatly wrapped in Christmas paper. I opened it to find a mug with a series of pictures of Fortune on it that depicted his progression from sick lamb to healthy adolescent sheep. It was full of chocolates, too. Sue, teary-eyed, hugged me warmly.

'You never gave up on the little guy,' she reminded me fondly. 'I thought you were going to say we needed to put him down and there wasn't any hope . . . and he was just a sheep after all . . .'

'I think it's clear Fortune isn't just a sheep, Sue. He's your little buddy!'

Fortune rubbed his head on Sue's leg impatiently.

'I'm going on a hunch and guessing you won't be having lamb for Christmas?' she asked, a twinkle in her eye.

I laughed. As it turned out, she was right. I had never been a vegetarian and had never dreamed of changing my diet, but eating lamb now quite simply didn't make sense to me. Spending each spring helping to save people's pet lambs had left me wondering if it was a more responsible choice to at least eat an adult animal.

I left hoping there wasn't going to be a sick turkey waiting for me back at the clinic. Christmas was only a few weeks away, after all.

CHAPTER TWENTY-FOUR

NOT ROITE

CHRISTMAS CAME AND WENT, and with it the dry heat of the Canterbury summer. As the New Zealand autumn brought misty hills and cool mornings, it occurred to me that another summer was just a plane ride away. I had heard intriguing tales of the English countryside from other vets, so, unable to resist, I flew to England before the first dusting of snow had touched our paddocks.

The mild summer afternoon drifted on as I wound my way up and down hills and through England's tiny southern villages. I passed the historical estates of old barons, long forgotten, surrounded by squat stone walls. They often featured ancient low-roofed stables, some of which were still in use. Cob houses made in centuries past were complete with thatched roofs sprouting stone chimneys.

The hedge-lined country lanes were so narrow that, despite my car being minuscule, whenever I encountered an oncoming vehicle a standoff would inevitably ensue. Eventually, one of us would have to reverse to a spot with enough room to allow the other to squeeze past. The operation involved a lot of gesturing and polite waves, and, on occasion, a stubborn stare that said, quite simply, 'I shall not yield.' The occasional elderly gardener would smile and wave at me as I drove by, searching for the country house where my next patient waited.

True summer was yet to arrive, and the hedges were still a deep green despite it being mid-June. I had been reliably informed that they did in fact have the occasional summer here in England, but I had yet to experience it myself.

As usual, that morning my GPS was proving to be useless. Apparently, these narrow lanes and old houses were the one thing left that Google hadn't wrapped its digital head around. Instead, I referred to my hurried scrawl on the torn page lying on the passenger seat.

> *Right at the church. If you hit Cobblesbridge, you've gone too far . . . 12 Milestone Hill . . . second lane on the left after the creek . . . there's a broken wall . . .*

I pulled over to where I was sure the house was meant to be, only to find myself staring into an empty field. A long-abandoned rusted tractor peered back at me with its one remaining eye. Blimey. I was lost. Again.

Getting lost had become an almost daily routine in the countryside's winding maze of high-sided hedged lanes. As I peered, and reversed, and craned my neck to try to work out where I was, I couldn't help wondering whether James Herriot had had the same navigation issues. Herriot's series of famous veterinary books, chronicling his work throughout the Yorkshire Dales in the 1930s through the 1950s, were an inspiration to me and many young vets alike.

If Herriot was still around to chat with, I'm sure he would have agreed that countryside house calls seem to go one of two ways. Scenario one: a growling German shepherd tries to eat you in a dank, musty room that smells of old boots. Scenario two: a fluffy kitten licks your hand in the faded but charming drawing room of an old manor, after which you are plied with scones and cups of tea. There didn't seem to be any middle ground.

I sincerely hoped this house call involved scones.

Ten minutes and a phone call back to the clinic later, I was bumping down a pot-holed track towards an old farmhouse. Drawing to a halt, I stepped out of the car and picked my way across a yard that was scattered with years of retired farm equipment. An old oak tree cast a dancing shadow on the grass. The air smelled of damp leaves and wet wood.

I knocked on the farmhouse's solid oak door and was let in by an old farmer. He led me to a simply furnished living room, where he deftly scooped up a little black cat that sat huddled on the couch. Popping her onto the dining table, he took a step back and pronounced, 'Not roite.'

I looked at the cat, then back at the farmer.

'She's not roite, she's not,' he repeated firmly in his thick, rolling West Country burr.

I waited to see whether more details would be forthcoming. They weren't. 'Uh right, okay . . . So what seems to be the problem with her?' I ventured.

'Not. Roite.'

'Have you noticed anything specific? Is she eating and drinking?' I pressed.

'Naw, she's ate nawt, and nawt drinkin neihver. Jus' sittin on th' porrch loike . . . Not roite, oiye say. Quwoite owt oh character for err.'

I peered at the cat, which sat quietly on the table watching us. She was breathing harder than was normal. 'Not quite breathing normally, is she?' I observed.

'Not roite! See!' he agreed. Then the old man paused in thought. 'Do ye fink shez got paints?'

'I'm sorry?'

'Paints. Do ye fink shez got paints?'

I had never heard of this condition. 'Paints?' I asked.

'Yer! Ya know loike, paints. Could she be havin' paints?'

My mind was racing to piece together what on earth he was talking about. Then, epiphany.

'Pains!' I exclaimed, as if I had just guessed the correct answer in a game of charades.

'Yer. Paints!' he echoed, jubilant that we were now on the same page.

'It's possible she is in pain; I'll take a look and see what we can find out. If only she could talk, huh? She could just tell us.'

'She'd tell us shez not roite, I'd say.'

We had agreed that she was not roite. After a thorough

examination, I concluded she was in pain, and likely had been injured on one of her recent adventures on the farm. Because of her breathing, I suggested we take an X-ray of her chest to make sure there were no fractures or issues with her lungs. I also suggested taking a blood sample to make sure something more serious wasn't affecting her.

'Sounds loike a gud plan tih me. When will ye tek it?'

'I can take her to the clinic and do it this afternoon,' I told him.

His eyebrows shot up. 'Yer a man o' action, you are! I loike it. Man o' action. Roite professional, that is. I can't fank ye enough, I can't.'

I couldn't help but smile at the farmer's effusive gratitude. It certainly wasn't the response I usually received at this point in the proceedings — usually, it was a somewhat uncomfortable conversation about the likely bill.

'Well, I guess you could say that . . . man of action, get it done, get it sorted. You know.' I grinned in spite of myself. My cheeks were starting to feel warm; jeez, was I blushing?

Embarrassed, I promptly turned to draw up some pain relief for the cat. Once I'd given her the injection, I scooped her up and eased her into the man's carrier cage.

Making it back to the clinic without getting lost, I took the cat into the X-ray room and took some shots. The images showed me that her chest was clear, and she had no broken bones.

While we ran her bloodwork in the machine, I watched her hunched up in the cage. Maybe it wasn't pain, maybe she was just sick. Her bloodwork came back with a slight increase in her white cell count, an indication of an inflammatory response somewhere in the body.

I needed more information. I took a drop of her blood, put it on a glass microscope slide, and used a second slide to spread the blood out along its surface into a thin film. Making a blood smear would allow me to examine the cells individually under the microscope. Once the blood was dry, I dipped it in a stain that dyes the cells, making them stand out for examination.

Many of her blood cells were filled with tiny purple dots that didn't belong there. The tiny dots were intracellular bacteria, an organism that lives within other cells, making it hard to kill. And if I were to have any chance of getting on top of it, I needed to find out exactly which bacteria it was.

Opening a pathology textbook, I found a picture that matched what I saw under the microscope. Anaplasma. A pathogen spread by ticks, something we are fortunate not to have in New Zealand. If left untreated, it could spread further and put the cat at serious risk. Thankfully, once diagnosed it's just a matter of putting the animal on the right antibiotic. I called the owner and advised that we would start the antibiotic and keep her overnight for supportive care.

The next morning, as I brought her outside to the farmer, who was waiting in the parking lot, she looked much brighter. He came briskly over and grasped my hand in a firm shake.

He regarded me warmly. 'Oiye be moch obloieged to yuwe, oiye be. Moch obloieged.' He went on to say a few more things, but I could not for the life of me tell you what they were.

When he had said his piece, I let him know that his little farm cat would be all right. I waved to him as he drove away, and caught him wiping a tear from his eye as he chatted to the cat in the carrier cage on the seat beside him.

I went back inside to find my next call ready and waiting.

CHAPTER TWENTY-FIVE

BISHOP'S CANNOCK

THE NEXT CALL WAS TO a small hilltop village called Bishop's Cannock. One of the clinic's clients, Mrs Scott, had a racehorse with a laceration on his leg. As I pulled around a corner, a vibrant green valley dotted with trees opened up before me. I found my turnoff and wound up a gravel drive before coming to a stop in front of a large stone cottage. As I climbed out of the car, a small elderly woman came striding out to greet me, shadowed by a little terrier.

'Hi, you must be Mrs Scott. How are you?' I asked cheerfully.

'I suppose this will cost me a fortune,' she replied, her clipped accent regal. 'Follow me, follow me,' she ordered, leaving the terrier to guard the house.

Mrs Scott took me across a hilly field to where a large brown ex-racehorse stood patiently in an aged wooden stable. His stall mate walked up, snuffling for food, but with a casual whack Mrs Scott flicked him aside so we could enter. We made our way over to the injured horse, which stood watching us quietly from the back of his dimly lit stall.

She pointed out a puncture wound above his right elbow. I walked the tall stallion out from the stall and into the sunlight so I could get a better look. The puncture wound was small, but deep. It was oozing pus, and his leg immediately below the wound was swollen with cellulitis. It was clear the wound needed flushing.

I made up a mixture of iodine and water in a metal dish and drew it up into a large syringe. With the needle still attached, I squirted a fine jet of the solution at the fleshy wound. The big stallion twitched his skin in response, irritated, and made to step away. Mrs Scott shot him a stern look and he stilled. I repeated this several times, flushing the wound as the stallion stamped his annoyance.

Judging the area adequately cleaned, I put some mānuka honey, something I have found works wonders for wound healing, over the site. I left the wound uncovered, as I've observed that leaving a smaller wound open to sunlight and air allows it to dry and heal faster. The honey also keeps flies from landing directly on the wound.

I counted out sachets of antibiotics and pain relief for Mrs Scott to mix into his feed. Her expression became increasingly grim as they piled up in her outstretched palms.

'More expense!' she complained.

'Unfortunately, he won't improve without it. Horses are expensive beasts,' I tried in my best conciliatory voice. Attempting to change the subject, I nodded towards her fine Victorian cottage. 'You have a beautiful house,' I said.

'You can buy it!' she replied.

'It's . . . for sale?' I asked, puzzled by her outburst.

'Well — look!' She pointed across the valley at the large, shiny corrugated iron building on the opposite hillside, as if this explained everything.

She pursed her lips. 'With *that* there, *my* place is next to worthless now. A Dutch *barn*, they call it. More like a monstrosity if you ask me. Just horrendous. Look at the thing! Bishop's Cannock is *NOT* a happy place,' she concluded with a sniff.

I raised an eyebrow, intrigued; then, on a whim, I decided to join her outrage. 'Bishop's Cannock is "up in arms", you could say?' I tempted.

'Bishop's Cannock is UP. IN. ARMS. INDEED!' Her voice increased in both pitch and volume. 'And that's not the worst of it!' She redirected my gaze to the roof of a house barely visible above the trees. 'Look over there!'

I struggled to see where she was pointing.

'No, no, down there — that *roff*. Look!' she insisted.

I looked.

'Some woman from Wayyyyles has had the *audacity* to move here and start a rrrookery!' She rolled the 'r' in 'rookery' for a remarkably long time.

'Wales!' I piped up in the best appalled tone I could muster. 'She's got a lot of nerve coming around here!'

'I have no idea how she got consent for it,' Mrs Scott grumbled. 'Matey-matey with the council no doubt. Those *things* are going to make a God-awful squawking racket once they hatch, I say!' she humphed breathlessly.

'Noisy rascals, those birds,' I agreed.

Beads of sweat were forming on her wrinkled forehead despite the cool breeze.

Feeling that things were beginning to escalate, I directed our conversation back to the issue at hand.

'Anyway,' I said with a sigh, 'that puncture wound is quite deep. I am going to need to come back and give him his tetanus jabs.'

Mrs Scott looked utterly defeated. 'More money! Oh Lord. I suppose if I don't, he will go and die on me, knowing my rotten bloody luck. Fine, fine. See you tomorrow.' And with that she dismissed me.

I admit, I felt a little relieved that her hands were occupied with holding the supply of horse's meds, otherwise I would not have put it past her to send me on my way with another of those casual whacks of the hand.

I hurried back to my car, simultaneously questioning the wisdom of stirring her up and revelling in the thrill of the lively exchange. Nothing quite like a good old-fashioned English village drama to spice up the afternoon.

A student was with me the following day as I pulled up Mrs Scott's steep driveway. I had briefed the student, of course, warning her that under no circumstances was she to mention the barn, the rookery, expenses, or Mrs Scott's house.

The sky was a clear blue, and the sun had a little heat in it. Summer might have finally arrived.

'Hi again!' I stepped out of the car to the greeting party of chatelaine and testy terrier.

'How are you today?' I asked foolishly.

'The lawn mower broke and it's too hot!' Mrs Scott huffed.

'Oh dear! A good excuse to put off seeing to it until tonight when it's cooler, eh?'

I paused, then gave into an impish urge, pitching my voice up to an inescapably baiting tone. 'Right about when the sun will be shimmering off that iron roof over there.'

My arm fell slowly as I aimed a finger at her hated Dutch friend across the valley.

The student stared at me, appalled. The results were instantaneous.

Her colour deepened to a deadly crimson. 'Oh, that *bloody* barn! HEINOUS and HORRENDOUS! But that's nothing. It's this damned rrrookery that really boils my blood! Birds. God! What a racket. As if Bishop's Cannock needs that!'

Glancing over the incensed woman's shoulder, I could see the student silently bobbing up and down, a hand clasped over her mouth, eyes watering. Mrs Scott was panting from the exertions of her rage. Her eyes glazed over as she drifted off to a distant place, no doubt imagining a violent feathery explosion across the valley.

Deciding I'd done enough damage, I ushered our little group over to where the horse was waiting.

With a note of satisfaction, I saw that the swelling had reduced. However, the wound itself continued to ooze thick yellow exudate. After cleaning it once more, I advised Mrs Scott to continue cleaning the wound as I had done, and to apply the mānuka honey.

He needed two tetanus injections. The first was an antitoxin to stop the immediate effects of the bacterial toxins. The second was a toxoid, which is an antigen that creates long-term tetanus immunity. I gave the antitoxin injection under the skin, then turned to Mrs Scott.

'Do you mind if the veterinary student gives the other tetanus injection?' I enquired.

Mrs Scott regarded the young woman, then turned back to give the horse's halter a sharp pull as he tossed his head impatiently. 'I don't care. As long as she doesn't jab me!' she said.

I chuckled and turned to face the student, who was frozen in fear.

I passed her the full syringe. 'Have you done this before?' I asked, shifting to a more practical tone.

'I haven't, no.' The huge racehorse towered over her.

The first time I'd given a horse an injection was in the Outback in Australia with five leather-skinned stockmen on horseback surrounding me like a panel of macho judges. It had been terrifying. In the more serene setting of the British countryside, I walked up to the horse, touched his neck and then rubbed it briskly. I grabbed a handful of skin over the muscled part of the neck, holding it firmly.

'They don't feel it as much if you do this,' I demonstrated. 'It's called a skin twitch. This injection needs to go into the muscle. Put the needle in just below where you're holding the skin; it should be perpendicular to the horse to make sure it goes deep enough. Push it all the way down into the muscle, then inject it.' I stepped back.

Mrs Scott watched curiously, still holding the horse. The student timidly stepped up beside the horse's neck, standing at his shoulder. She gently grabbed some skin.

'Grab it like you mean it!' The impatient Australian vet's tone was in my mouth. Catching myself, I continued more softly. 'The skin twitch only works properly if you take more of the skin and hold it firmly.'

She grabbed a bigger handful of skin. With a shaky hand, she prodded the needle into the horse. He lifted his head, his eyes widening. Mrs Scott tugged on the rope, pulling his head down once more. The student pressed the plunger, emptying it to complete the injection.

'Well done,' I praised. 'Mrs Scott might just let you have the first bid on her house — it's up for sale, you know.'

The student looked baffled, while the corner of Mrs Scott's mouth twitched with the ghost of a grin. As we packed up and made our way back to the car, I pictured the dreaded baby birds cracking their way out of their eggs, oblivious to the fact that they were hatching into a war zone.

Mrs Scott marched ahead of us as we crossed the lush field, stands of trees at its edges. The horse's halter swung from her hand as she strode along. I feared for the Dutch, the Welsh, and anyone else with ambitions for that valley. Bishop's Cannock was up in arms indeed!

CHAPTER TWENTY-SIX

JACARÉ

I DUG DEEP WITH MY OAR, happy to put space between me and all of the people. The paddleboard sliced the murky water, leaving gentle ripples in its wake. Twisted mangroves lined the edges of the waterway, leaning to watch as I passed below.

I was taking a break from animals to do some work for the church in Brazil. The hostel I was staying at was on a small island nestled among the mangroves of Rio de Janeiro. The water beneath my board was muddy; moments earlier I had seen a nappy floating past. A fall into it would leave me with a skin infection if I was lucky, giardia if I wasn't. Nevertheless, I was confident in my paddleboarding skills, dodging the boats that whipped back and forth across the waterway, buffeting me with their wake.

This confidence was not necessarily shared by the locals. Indeed, the hostel owner had looked decidedly concerned when he spotted me digging out the cobweb-covered paddleboard from behind the building.

'Are you sure?' he'd asked anxiously. 'There's a lot of boats — you could get run over.'

'I can manage them,' I'd replied. 'Anything else? Anacondas, piranhas, 'gators?' I'd teased.

'Just be careful of the boats: they won't slow down for you.'

He hadn't lied. In fact, the shirtless captains of the narrow powerboat ferries sped up as they passed, laughing as they tried to send me toppling. So far, I had dodged their menacing and kept out of the toxic sludge.

'Jacaré!' a ferryman called out, smiling as he shot past in his sleek wooden boat. I angled my board towards his incoming wake and bent my knees, balancing as I crested the waves. What does 'jacaré' mean? I wondered as I paddled on.

There was a lull in the ferry activity, so I paddled to my right and turned off the main channel into a smaller one. The sounds of boats faded, and the melody of birds and insects took over. It was a clear day, aside from the column of smoke that drifted up from a small bushfire atop one of the mountains overlooking the mangroves. I gazed around to look for the statue of Christ the Redeemer; it was nowhere to be seen. The tangled roots of the trees that lined the channel dipped into the water, drinking. It was nice to finally get away from all the noise and hustle of the busy city.

What's more, I had some pondering to do. The day before, my friend had mentioned a certain 'special lady' whom he was convinced was the perfect match for me. He knew her from his hometown in Finland. He'd shown me a picture of her, and she was breathtaking, stunning and gorgeous all at once. The only minor problem was that she lived in Finland. Still . . .

Back on the water, I was following that appealing train of thought when the discordant cry of a bird brought me back to the here and now. I realised that it had been a good while since I had seen a boat or any human life at all.

I glanced down once more at the stagnant water below. Could anything live in this murk? Then I noticed a strange-looking log, sitting on the surface near one of the trees at the bank. I paddled over to investigate. The log vanished.

Horror swept over me. I thrust my paddle in the water, dragging it to stop my forward momentum, turning away from the spot so recently vacated by the nimble 'log'. My heart began to thump in my chest. I cautiously examined another spot in the water under the tree roots. With dismay, I realised a similar dark shape was protruding from the surface, watching me . . .

Jacaré — *alligator!*

My throat went dry as I paddled onward. I hoped that disturbing the water as little as possible would grant me respite from an attack.

Moments later I came upon an open, muddy bank. On it were half a dozen or so alligators, each as long as I was tall, lying like statues in the sun — but they weren't motionless for long. Their eyes flicked open at my appearance, and then the congregation moved as one, clawing down the bank towards the water to slither in. They glided towards me, tails swishing back and forth.

I froze. Panic tightened my chest. My pulse whooshed in my ears, and my hearing seemed to dull, making the sounds of the jungle muted, indistinct and strange. Any thoughts of the sultry Scandinavian, the day, my memories . . . everything retreated, until all that remained was me and this pack of ancient reptiles.

They swam halfway between the shore and my paddleboard, then dipped below the surface, out of sight. My heart rate ratcheted up another notch. There were at least seven or eight alligators under me. With horror, I realised that they didn't care who I was, or what kind of life I had led. They ran on primal instincts. If their stomachs told them to eat, they would eat. If I lost my nerve and fell from the board, they would think I was some animal falling into the water and tear me apart.

Then the awful reality hit me: if I fell, I *was* some animal falling in the water.

My whole body was as taut as a twisted rope. I kept my knees bent, the nose of my board pointed deeper into the channel, as I coasted further from the main lagoon and the boats. How I missed those boats! I didn't dare stop and turn around, because that would risk disturbing the water — or worse, provide the toothed creatures below with a chance to bump the board.

I was astonished by how utterly vulnerable I had

become, shirtless and with nothing but a thin layer of fibreglass between me and their deadly jaws. I carefully paddled on as fast as I could without splashing, hoping to get away, hoping they wouldn't knock my board and send me tumbling into the water.

I looked back cautiously, careful not to lose my balance. There was no sign of activity on the water's surface. I paddled on, barely remembering to breathe. I was paddling further away from civilisation, on top of which, the channel was narrowing. I stopped as I saw the channel close into a thick wall of roots and branches: a dead end.

A bird burst out from under a bush overhanging the water. Startled, I jumped, wobbling on the board.

I wanted to deny that this was happening, to complain about the unfairness of it all. An hour earlier I had been enjoying a cold drink in a hammock — and now this! My mind couldn't process it . . . couldn't evaluate, think calmly or rationally, or plot.

This time, it was *my* instinct's turn to kick in.

I started slowing the board down, hesitantly turning it around to head back.

Back.

Past the alligators.

I was considering climbing from the board up into the trees, and then trekking back to town barefoot, when a harsh screech came from the jungle.

I crouched down on the board.

'What now?' I demanded of the mangroves.

Something large was crashing through the bush.

I looked over to see a grey-brown animal the size of a pig smashing through the trees, running away from something. A long snout hung down the front of its face.

'A tapir? Maybe that's what these alligators will think I am when they eat me,' I muttered. With that, I resolved to return the way I came. Alligator Avenue. I started to paddle; I started to pray.

'I'm too young to be eaten,' I whispered.

I was paddling as fast as I could without splashing. The board drifted forward, a V of ripples trailing behind me. I approached the small muddy bank, streaked with the footprints and belly marks of the 'gators' entry. They were nowhere to be seen. I held my breath, forcing myself to stop imagining one leaping up at me.

I was past it. I paddled on, but didn't begin to relax until the sound of boats filled my ears again. How I now welcomed the danger of being flattened by the zooming vessels. Anything was better than being torn apart by alligators.

Once I was back in relatively open water, what had just happened felt oddly surreal, as if it had happened to someone else. Would anyone believe me? It didn't matter. What mattered was that I was still alive, with a full complement of limbs, and that my little impromptu ecology tour had come to an end.

Two weeks later I was sitting on a small grassy knoll in a park outside my old Bible school in Northern California, letting the sun warm my face. As I sat basking, I was still processing my surprise at receiving a message from my Finnish friend telling me that the mysterious woman in the picture he'd shown me was in California, too. She had landed a few days after I had, and, what's more, she was visiting the same town I was in today. I'd asked him for her number, but he'd told me she was the type of woman who would run a mile if some guy she didn't know asked to meet up with her. So I guessed that if we were to meet, it would have to be in God's hands.

Still, it wouldn't hurt to give the odds a little nudge now, would it? He'd mentioned in passing that she would probably visit the school as she'd talked about wanting to go there some day, and, besides, there wasn't exactly that much else to see or do in this little town. Which is why I was now waiting outside, idly peeling a blade of grass in half, instead of going straight into class.

As I watched the students trickling into the building, chatting happily, I noted she wasn't among them. I sighed, dejected. The odds were clearly resisting my nudge.

'Just "bump" into her?' I muttered to no one in particular. This was ridiculous. I needed to head into class before they shut the doors on me.

As I reached over for my bag, something caught my eye. A figure was walking onto the field in the distance . . . Squinting against the sun, I could just make out a flash of golden hair and a white dress, moving in the wind. As she crossed the park, her features sharpened. Could this be her?

Before I could decide for sure, she had passed by and had entered the building. I'd been so transfixed that I had forgotten to time my entrance! If I didn't hurry, she'd be sitting with some olive-oil Californian guy by the time I got in.

I hurried to the door and was relieved to see that the mystery woman was still in the auditorium, getting a visitor sticker. She was leaning over the desk, writing, and I still couldn't make out her face. I hurriedly ripped my own visitor sticker off and screwed it into a ball as I went back over to the sign-in desk. The woman at the desk looked at me quizzically.

'I lost it,' I shrugged, reaching for a fresh sticker. I put it down on the table next to the mystery woman.

'Hi there,' I ventured casually.

'Hello,' she replied, her voice as warm as honey. But as lovely as she was, I was disappointed. It wasn't her. This woman had a British accent.

Still, there was no harm in chatting to a nice woman now that I had started, so I carried on.

'Oh, so are you from England?' I asked her.

'England?' she laughed easily. 'No, I'm from Finland.'

With that, I glanced up and she did the same.

It was her. My composure was a piece of glass, shattered but not quite broken; I barely held it together.

'Fin— Finland?' I managed. Her hair was like sun-kissed wheat. Her intense blue-green eyes held my gaze.

I fumbled my way through some small talk. I was an ungainly boy trying to scoop a butterfly from a leaf without it dancing away. I couldn't just tell her I knew who she was, could I?

Finally, we mutually 'discovered' that we had a friend in common, then laughed at the remarkable coincidence.

I invited her to sit with me, so we sat. I invited her to dinner, and we ate. Then to a beautiful river to soak in the thermal springs. We laughed, and then we kissed. Emboldened, I asked her to forget Finland for the moment and fly back to New Zealand with me. We flew.

Ten months later, atop a small mountain, I asked her to marry me.

CHAPTER TWENTY-SEVEN

THE MIDDLE EAST

'WHAT THE HELL!?' Anna screamed, pressing her hands against the car roof.

The car slammed down on the road at 100 kilometres per hour, the suspension bottoming out with a grinding crunch. On our left, the sun was dipping behind rocky mountains. To our right, a blue desert lake created by the spring rains shimmered in the evening light. It would have been the perfect evening if it hadn't been punctuated by these airborne episodes.

'You need to *slow down*,' Anna said through gritted teeth.

I had been hoping to get to the village before dark, but this was looking less and less likely. The judder bars on the highway were enormous, and unmarked — they blended seamlessly with the road. I was already dreading returning our rental car; the rear bumper was hanging by a thread.

On either side of the road, the sandy ground held a smattering of shrubs. Ahead, a line of camels approached. To Anna's relief, I slowed down to a crawl.

They were strange to look at, enormous and elegant with long, spindly legs. I opened the window and one of the camels stopped, dipping her head down to stick her long nose through the window into my open palm. She sniffed and mouthed my hand, peering at us from beneath long, curled eyelashes. I had never realised how beautiful camels were. She moved on to join her herdmates, and they continued to plod down the middle of the highway on wide, padded feet.

The camels were why I was here. Following the emergence of the Covid-19 pandemic, camels had become a particular subject of interest because they harboured a similar coronavirus. This virus was also zoonotic — meaning it could spread from animals (in this case, camels) to humans — and could cause serious symptoms, even death. I had joined a team conducting field research to establish the prevalence of MERS (Middle East respiratory syndrome) in both camels and humans in the Middle East. It was hoped that our work could not only reduce the prevalence and transmission of MERS, but also provide some valuable insights into the behaviour of zoonotic coronaviruses.

We continued for another 20 minutes, passing small villages with squat cinderblock buildings, leaving the lake behind.

'Here's good,' Anna said, pointing off the highway to a dirt track leading up a small rise.

I pulled off the road and we hopped out of the car. It was surprisingly cool. Although it was early spring, I'd assumed it would be hot year-round in the desert. Anna passed me her camera and gave me a list of instructions for the cover shot of the album she was recording. She'd found a seemingly perfect location — and an inept photographer.

She stood at the top of the sand dune, her white dress billowing in the wind, framed by red-brown mountains in a scene bathed with golden light. I still couldn't believe this stunning Scandinavian was my wife. In between snapping pictures, I noticed a collection of buildings, about half a kilometre away, between us and the mountains. Something wasn't right about the scene, but I couldn't put my finger on it. I took a few more photos, then stopped and looked again at the compound.

'What are you doing? We are losing the light,' Anna said.

I examined the buildings. Far away though they were, I could make out a long, narrow building and a water tower.

'I think we should leave,' I said, beginning to feel uneasy.

'What's the problem? Take a few more shots, then we can go.'

'No, no — let's go.' I moved quickly down the rise towards the car, Anna following reluctantly. I handed her the camera, walked over to the car and got in.

We had been married less than a year, and in that time had lived in New Zealand and then Finland, and had just moved to the Middle East. The pace of change had been exciting, but was also a lot to take in. We had started learning Arabic months before arriving, but I had a feeling it was nowhere near enough.

Now, I heard a rumbling behind the car, and turned to see armed troops piling out of a military truck. A massive

50-calibre gun was mounted on the back, a soldier arming it. My stomach went into my throat as soldiers surrounded the car. I put down my window and looked for Anna. To my astonishment she had her face in the camera, and was pointing it at her sandals.

'Anna!'

She looked up, her mouth forming an 'o' of surprise.

'Get in the car!' I called.

The soldiers let her past, and she climbed into the passenger seat beside me.

The officer in charge was at my window. 'Taab,' he said, holding out his hand.

I had no idea what it meant, but I handed over our passports, assuming that's what he wanted. I glanced nervously at the soldiers' guns as they stood around our car.

He passed our passports back to another soldier, who walked back to the truck with them. That didn't feel promising. He pointed at the camera in Anna's hands, speaking a stream of Arabic. Again, I didn't catch a single word, but I gave him the camera, too. He passed it to another trooper, who began looking through the photos. The men began a rapid exchange, gesturing and pointing at the camera.

Soldier one turned his attention to me and asked a question in Arabic. I understood nothing. Those lessons were useless! He didn't seem to be using any of the words I had learned.

'I can't speak Arabic,' I told him.

He continued, and began to get frustrated. Turning to

his squad mates, he gave an order, and two of them went back to the truck and drove off.

'You . . . wait,' he said, pointing at me.

We sat for a long time as the soldiers looked through the pictures. I began to wonder what it would be like in a military prison. Whether we would get a trial or even be allowed a phone call. Whether we would ever get our passports back. Would we be deported? This was either going to be the shortest work trip of my life, or — worse — the longest.

Anna and I sat in silence, deciding it was better not to talk in English and potentially cause further problems.

Finally, the truck came back. A pair of soldiers approached, one of them new. He came over and spoke with the officer before looking at the camera.

He turned to me. 'You can't be here.' He pointed at the camera. 'Very bad, no no no.'

'I'm sorry, we're tourists. I didn't know.' I was grateful Anna was with me, looking as innocent as a human could look in her white dress and make-up.

He pointed in the direction of the buildings. 'Military base.'

It was all starting to make sense — they thought we were photographing their base. Luckily, I had kept the buildings out of the shots, a vague instinct telling me that the buildings might be military.

A soldier finished looking through the photos, then said something in Arabic. Remarkably, I understood.

'The pictures are all of her,' he said. A soldier chuckled, and I felt the tension break.

The soldier who knew English made a gesture towards those in the truck, then turned back to us and spoke again. 'You go now. Never come here again, understand?' He took our passports, which a soldier had just brought over, and handed them back to us.

I nodded emphatically. 'Yes, of course. We are very sorry.'

The truck rumbled back so we could pass. I reversed and pulled back onto the highway before they could change their minds. I was relieved to be driving away, like someone who had just slipped the noose.

'You looked so ridiculous photographing your feet when they arrived . . . I think that's probably what saved us,' I said.

Anna shook her head in disbelief. 'I wonder what would have happened if the base was in the background of a phot— Hey, look!' Anna was pointing at a towering fence in the distance on our right. Behind it was an airbase, large military aircraft taxiing down the runway.

We drove on as the desert faded into darkness. Ahead was a checkpoint, and the ute in front of us slowed and stopped to talk to an officer. After a few seconds, the ute moved on and I pulled up.

An Arabic man with a short beard leaned forward and looked at us. 'Welcome! Where from?'

'New Zealand,' I gestured at Anna, 'and Finland.'

'Ahlan wa Sahlan,' he said, waving us through.

'After that last incident I thought we were in for something much less casual than that,' Anna said, the relief clear in her voice.

'I think if you're just being normal and not wandering around military bases with your camera, you're generally fine,' I replied, laughing.

The truth was I did feel nervous, though. I had never been to the Middle East before, and now we were moving here for the year.

Passing another airport, I was surprised to see Humvees flanking the runway, facing out towards the highway. Little blue alternating lights blinked from their hoods. The line of them seemed to never end as we drove along.

I counted 30 before I turned to Anna. 'I guess some military general is arriving?'

'I doubt we will ever know,' she said.

'There's a war zone on pretty much every side of the border, so I imagine this is just the norm here.'

When we finally pulled into the village, I was surprised to see how busy it was. The streets were well lit, and on either side of the road were cafés and restaurants where men sat together drinking tea and smoking shisha.

A guy stepped out in front of our car and I slammed on the brakes, almost running him over. He looked at me, confused, and crossed in front of us. A little shocked, I drove on, but didn't get more than 50 metres before it happened again. This time I stopped before the man had taken more than a few steps onto the road.

‘I think pedestrians have right of way . . .’ Anna pointed out.

The village was a hive of activity: all the shops were open, and people were sitting at outdoor tables eating chicken and rice from a huge shared plate.

We found a restaurant and sat down to eat.

The server came over. ‘Welcome!’ he said.

Everyone said ‘Welcome’. I loved it.

After we had eaten I went to pay, but my card didn’t work. Far from being perturbed, our host just waved me away, saying, ‘No problem. You come back and pay tomorrow. You are welcome!’

The next day I went to the office to meet the project’s lead vet, Hans. He was sitting at a desk, pipetting liquid from a brown glass bottle into little plastic pottles. I picked up a pipette to help as we talked. A drop of the liquid landed on my trousers.

‘This stuff isn’t dangerous, is it? I just dropped some on my pants,’ I said.

Hans picked up the bottle to read the label. ‘It doesn’t say it’s corrosive. It’s the viral medium that we store the camel nasal samples in, so in theory it shouldn’t be too destructive . . .’

Hans explained the plan for the week. We would be heading into the desert to sample several camel herds. As he spoke, I began to smell something strange. A thread of smoke coiled up from my trousers. I leapt up, sending my chair toppling backwards, and frantically pulled down my pants, kicking them off across the room. I stood in my underwear, panting.

Hans was staring at me with a disturbed look on his face. I pointed across the room at my trousers, trying to get my words in order.

'The pants, it was the pants.'

Hans was likely regretting his hiring decision. I went over to the scrunched-up trousers and carefully unravelled them. There was a burn hole where the fluid had landed.

I spent the rest of the morning sitting in my underwear. When a local woman came in, Hans had to hide me in a cupboard until she left. It was a relief when Hans's wife arrived with a spare pair of trousers.

Three days later I was driving through the desert with Hans, searching for a shepherd called Abu Ahmed. We had entered through a minor checkpoint in the mountains that was used only by the Bedouin. Hans had spoken to the checkpoint guards in fluent Arabic, while I nodded along, oblivious to the details.

I had been surprised when Hans told me I could take the wheel. When he'd asked if I could drive on sand, I'd said yes. I'd driven on the beach once, and figured that was qualification enough.

Now the ute felt as if it was gliding as we flew along,

passing towering red rock formations. Some were vast and wide like sleeping animals, others jutted up like crashed spacecraft lodged in the sand. They could have been a thousand dusty pancakes stacked to the sky. Water had eaten away at the surface of the rock, leaving it with innumerable streaks and holes. Wind-blown sand piled at their feet.

I'd assumed the desert would be lifeless and barren, but it was far from it. It was spring. Tiny purple flowers sprouted from the sand, whole colourful areas of desert stretching out like a royal carpet. In the distance, a jagged mountain range was silhouetted against the haze.

I drove over a rise and slowed down. In front of us a Bedouin herdsman was leading a flock of sheep, his staff in hand. He was the second we had come across, the first directing us east. Beside him plodded a donkey with bags hanging from its saddle. The three dogs trotting on the outskirts of the flock eyed us with curiosity as I pulled up to stop on a firm patch of sand.

'As-salaam-alaikum,' the shepherd greeted us as we stepped from the ute.

The man wore a long brown robe and his head was wrapped with a white shemagh, a headscarf. His shepherd's staff had a crook for catching sheep.

'Wa-alaikum-salaam,' Hans replied, taking the shepherd's hand.

I followed suit. The shepherd said his name was Abu Mohammad, and, after Hans told him we were vets, he began to gesture to one of his sheep. Her udder was hanging low, but she looked bright enough otherwise.

'What's he saying?' I asked Hans.

'The sheep has a problem with her udder. We need to catch her and take a look.'

Together the three of us caught the sheep, and I flipped her onto her back. These sheep were nothing like the sheep back in New Zealand: they had fine, shaggy wool, well suited to the desert. I felt the sheep's udder and found no heat or swelling. I took her temperature; it was normal.

'It's not mastitis,' I said. 'I think the ligaments have gone.' Sometimes in older sheep the ligaments that support and hold up the udder can become overly stretched.

Hans passed on the diagnosis to the shepherd, and explained that she wouldn't be suitable for breeding in the future as she would struggle to feed the lambs. Hans then asked him for directions to Abu Ahmed, who owned a herd of camels. Our goal was to meet him and take blood and nasal samples from the herd.

We had been travelling through the desert like this for two hours, stopping whenever we saw herdsmen to get directions to Abu Ahmed's last known location. The GPS coordinates we had originally been using to find him had taken us to an old camp that looked as though it had been abandoned months before. Apparently, it was normal to track down the sampling herds like this. They moved all the time.

We drove on, arcing around a towering rock formation before dropping down a steep sand dune. Ahead was a lone dark canvas tent. As we pulled closer, I could see the tent was made of woven animal hair.

'It's made from goats' hair,' Hans explained when he saw me looking.

The tent was the size of a minibus and looked as though it could sleep at least 10 people.

Abu Ahmed greeted us, then put a large iron kettle directly on the fire outside the tent. He waved us inside while he stayed outside to tend to it. We sat waiting on a patterned rug. The gloom was a relief from the intense light of the desert and it was surprisingly cool. A canvas wall divided the tent in two. From the other side of the canvas, I heard a whisper and shuffling. I looked at Hans, but before I could ask any questions, Abu Ahmed returned with the steaming kettle and two small cups.

He poured the tea and passed us each a cup. Hans gulped the contents of his cup down in a few mouthfuls. I went to do the same, and almost choked. The tea tasted like pure sugar. Hans grinned knowingly. While he was talking about family in Arabic, Hans noticed I had barely touched my tea, and gestured at me to hurry up and drink it. I gathered it was rude not to, so I drank it down before we moved outside to find the camels.

They were scattered around the area, grazing on bushes. Abu Ahmed caught a large male, and clipped a rope to his halter. The bull camel was much larger than the females I'd seen on the highway, another few feet on top of what was already impossibly big. I was supposed to blood-sample him?

Abu Ahmed made a long sound with his throat that resembled a wild cat's growl. The camel threw his head back stubbornly. He opened his mouth, drawing back his lips to reveal 7.5-centimetre canine teeth. The towering creature roared, his throat vibrating from the force. Chewed plant material came up and spurted from his mouth, a stinking torrent of green sludge.

The camel was like a dragon dragged from its cave. There was no way the old man could subdue the beast. I wondered if there was something I could do. I'd never imagined camels to be so bloody angry.

Finally, the bull camel knelt, and then sat, roaring the whole time. I put on a mask, took out a long needle and syringe, and approached as the camel watched me with a wide eye. As I drew near, he pulled his head around hard, making Abu Ahmed stumble. The camel was now facing me, roaring his displeasure. Stomach contents flew at my face, but I sidestepped just in time, avoiding the worst of it. It was like trying to hold a snake, one with the head of an oversized wolf. Not only that, but he had a slime cannon at his disposal. I was undeniably outgunned.

Hans came around to help Abu Ahmed with the rope. With the two of them handling the bull camel's head, I was able to get within jabbing range. I pressed down on his jugular with my left hand, and a vein the size of a hose-pipe popped up along his neck. I leaned forward and put the needle in, and the camel surged, getting to his feet fast, his big shoulder knocking me backwards. I regained my balance and looked down to see how much blood

I'd collected. There was a single drop in the syringe. It wouldn't do.

Hans had shown me how to take a sample on a docile female camel in the rocky valley close to the village. This was proving to be a completely different experience.

After another struggle, we got the camel sitting again. This time Abu Ahmed tied the camel's front feet together, wrapping the rope from one foot over the shoulders to the other. I tentatively approached once more, trying to keep my focus on the neck rather than his large teeth.

'When you block the vein, grab a handful of skin at the same time and brace against him so that when his neck moves, you move with him,' Hans instructed, still holding the rope tight.

It was sound advice. After the needle went in, the camel lurched his neck sideways. Now firmly braced against his neck, I could step with him, drawing back the syringe to finally get a sample. Relief. Job done.

But just as I began to relax, I saw Hans pulling a long cotton bud from his pocket, which he then passed to me. I'd forgotten about the nasal sample. I wouldn't have thought it possible, but the camel was more enraged now than when we had started. Getting a cotton bud in his nose looked about as likely as winning a grappling match with a dinosaur.

Abu Ahmed saw the cotton bud, and fast as a mongoose he struck, catching the camel by the nose. Stunned, the camel continued to roar but didn't throw his head. This allowed me to step forward, put the cotton bud in, spin it and take it out. I passed the bud back to Hans, and he snapped off the tip, putting it into a little plastic pottle containing the pants-eating liquid.

'As easy as that, huh?' I said to Hans, brushing camel stomach contents off my shirt.

'You still need to microchip him,' Hans said.

Another battle with the head ensued as I tried to jab the bull camel in the shoulder and he tried to swing around and bite me. Thankfully, I won.

Once more I thought our ordeal was over, only for Hans to hand me a scanner: I had to go back into the camel's biting radius and scan the chip, making sure it came up on the machine.

We carried on, working from camel to camel. Abu Ahmed's brother, Mahamoud, and Mahamoud's cousins, came to join us as the light faded. We were on the final camel, and I was grateful to be finishing for the day.

Mahamoud made the familiar guttural rasping sound and pulled on the rope. The camel sat, but then she lurched forward onto her feet once more. As she did, her head went forward and smashed into Mahamoud's forehead, teeth-first. He staggered back, crying out in shock. A thin trail of blood ran down his face, and he put a hand to his head. Hans and I took him to the side and cleaned the cut.

Mahamoud's cousins crowded around him, shouting in

Arabic. I had no idea what was going on, and, before I could ask Hans, they were all piling into an old ute and driving away.

'Where are they going?' I asked, as we packed the last of the samples into the cold box.

'To the medical centre in town,' Hans said.

'All of them?' I asked.

Hans nodded.

Abu Ahmed came over and spoke for a long while to Hans, gesturing in the direction of the ute disappearing in the distance and then towards his tent.

Hans translated for me. 'He says that people should always come first, and his family is his life. Glory to God because I am still alive to see my grandchildren grow and, God willing, I will have more years with my wives and children. Oh, and he invites us to come eat at his tent.'

Hans accepted the invitation, and we went back with Abu Ahmed to eat. As we approached the tent, I saw a woman, her head and face wrapped, disappear through the canvas flap on the far side. That explained the shuffling sound I'd heard earlier on the other side of the partition; it was the women's side.

Abu Ahmed produced a large bowl filled with what looked like bread mashed up with milk. His sons arrived in a beat-up, flat-bed ute to join us. Everyone began putting their hands into the bowl, balling up the mash and eating. As I began to follow suit Hans caught my hand before it reached the food. The boys covered their mouths, laughing.

'Other hand,' he said quietly.

I sheepishly withdrew my left hand and dug in with my right, vowing to learn the customs quickly so I didn't keep looking like an ass. (Later, he explained that the left hand is traditionally associated with toileting, and so it is taboo to use for handling food.)

We sat and talked for hours, drinking tea as the stars came out. At some point the cousins returned with Mahamoud, a neat strip of bandage covering the cut on his forehead. I had started more Arabic classes since arriving, but other than the odd word I understood little. It didn't seem to matter, and one of the teenage boys even put an arm around my shoulder warmly as we talked.

By the time we returned to the truck, a vibrant sky full of stars sprawled out above us. It was so vivid that I froze in place, staring up in awe. Despite the absence of the moon, the desert was lit by pale-white light.

'The stars are so bright they light up the whole desert!' I said, turning to Hans.

'Some of the things here I've gotten used to, but I'll never get used to this,' Hans replied.

I felt tiny, a speck in the sand below an endless cosmos.

We drove for half an hour until we found a good spot to set up camp. We didn't need much, just a rocky outcrop for a windbreak and a flat piece of sand. I fell asleep counting shooting stars, wondering if I was the luckiest vet on earth.

That first trip was the beginning of months of excursions into the surrounding desert. We worked high on the cliffs, looking down at ancient tombs and elaborate temples carved into the rock. Tourists milled along the paths below. I was grateful to be working with the locals rather than buying trinkets from them along the path.

Things were going well, and we found a rhythm after a slow start, sampling enough camels each week to hit our targets. Nurses came with us to take blood samples from the families working with the camels. We conducted questionnaires, with the goal of connecting specific farming practices with disease prevalence in both camels and humans.

One morning I arrived at the office to find Hans with his head in his hands.

'What's going on?' I asked.

'We're out of money,' he said.

'We can't be out of money; we have a massive budget.'

'It's not the budget.'

I stared at him, dumbfounded.

He went on. 'The money comes from the university in Europe, and funnels through the university here. The funnel is blocked.'

'What are you talking about?'

'They won't release the money for us to pay our nurses, our local vet or the rent for this office.'

'They can't just block the money, it's not theirs! How can they?' I objected.

'I got an email saying our paperwork isn't in order.'

I began to pace up and down the office. 'Let's drive to the university now and let them have it!'

Hans held up a placating hand. 'This sort of thing is normal — I'll sort it.'

Weeks passed, and several meetings later the money remained plugged. We were falling behind and getting calls from the landlord, who was upset about not getting his rent. As our sampling ground to a standstill, and with the work showing no sign of restarting soon, Anna and I decided we would have to move on and head home.

As we packed up our apartment, I found out that the man in charge of the local side of our project had put forward his own team and Hans was being replaced. All of the years Hans had spent building the project seemed to count for nothing.

It was a sad ending to an amazing project, but knowing its positive impact on the lives of thousands of Bedouin living in remote parts of the desert helped to soften the blow. Veterinary care, health care, medicine and hygiene supplies made a tangible difference to the families the project had visited.

The project revealed that the potentially dangerous virus was indeed present in the area. As a result, preventative measures are being suggested to the local camel herdsmen, such as handwashing before eating and wrapping their shemagh across their faces while working with young camels. The significance of the virus and its impact on world health is yet to be seen, and research on the disease is ongoing. I hope there will be many more projects like it in the future, where data gathering is combined with bringing important health care and aid to remote areas.

Surprisingly, the camel wasn't added to the long list of the ones that bit me. Maybe I'd finally picked up a few of the tricks I'd admired in my veterinary role models all those years ago.

I was blown away by the hospitality and kindness of the locals while we lived in the Middle East. They went out of their way to make us feel welcome, and their love for children and family was beautiful to see.

There's an Arabic expression, 'You can never cross the ocean unless you have the courage to leave sight of the shore.' When I heard it, I thought of all the richness that had been added to my life through the different places I'd visited and the special people I'd met — none of which could have happened without the uncomfortable sensation of stepping into the unknown.

The flip side of all the adventure was that I hadn't laid down any roots of my own yet, which is something I wanted to do as Anna and I looked to start our own family. But as another Arabic saying goes, 'The best time to plant a tree is twenty years ago. The second-best time is today.' I was heading home. Home, and ready for the next chapter of the veterinary adventure.

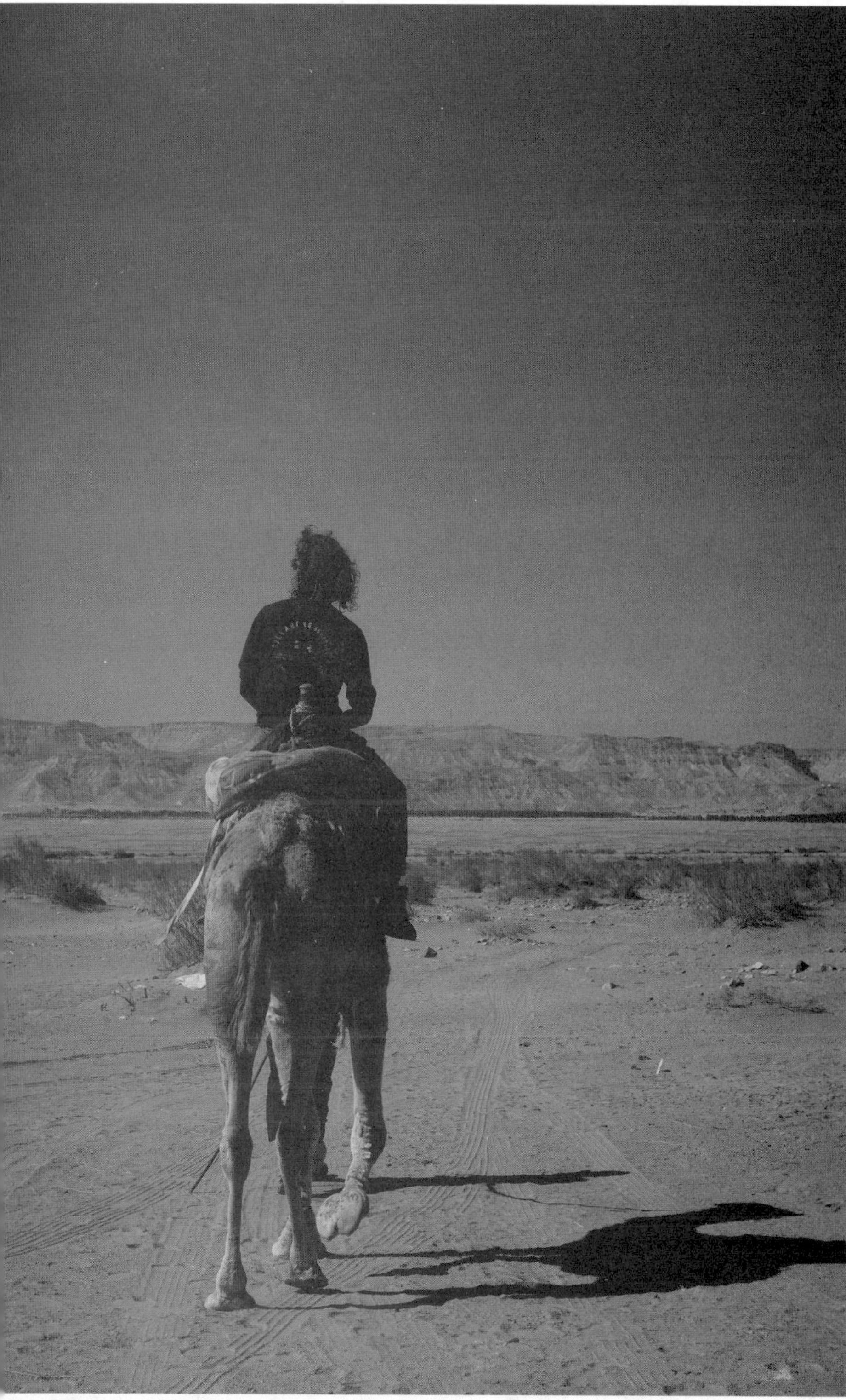

AFTERWORD

I AM STILL LEARNING what it means to be a good veterinarian, and I find myself forever facing new challenges and hurdles. Perhaps the biggest most recent challenge has been this project, which is as much a story about the life of a vet as it was an exercise in pouring myself onto the page.

Through my work I've learned how connected the lives of animals are with the people surrounding them. If a farmer cares for his stock, then they're well fed and sheltered and their ailments are cared for. If a pet owner loves their pet, the animal lives well. How locals care for their environment has a major impact on wildlife. If a country values the welfare of animals, they have well-trained vets and a system to protect them; if they don't, animals suffer. More than anything, the wellbeing of animals is up to us as individuals. We are undoubtably their stewards. If you or someone you know wants to become a vet, I would strongly advise spending time seeing the day-to-day realities of clinical practice first. It is often very different to what people expect, and it takes a great deal of resiliance and grit.

Whatever your passion, I believe that you should never stop pursuing knowledge and moving forward in your field. It's the gritty, unfamiliar things in life that bring us the smoothest finish.

ACKNOWLEDGEMENTS

I WOULD LIKE TO ACKNOWLEDGE my first editor, Dionne M., who helped get the book up to standard, and my second, Kate Stone, who polished the story wonderfully.

I would also like to give special thanks to my sister, Jo, my wife, Anna, and my mother, Catherine, who all poured a huge amount of time into helping me initially edit the book, and to Eddy, who helped me with my submission to publishers.

I'm deeply grateful, too, for all of the pilot readers who gave helpful feedback, especially Esther, Tamsin, Mrs Leggat, Mark, and my father, Jan.

I would also like to express my heartfelt thanks to Nadine Rubin Nathan and Anna Jackson-Scott for the support they provided, and to Emily Goldthorpe and designer Sarah Elworthy. Thanks as well to Matthew Buckingham for allowing his dog, Albi, to feature on the cover!

Finally, I extend my appreciation to the team at Massey University Press for believing in this book.

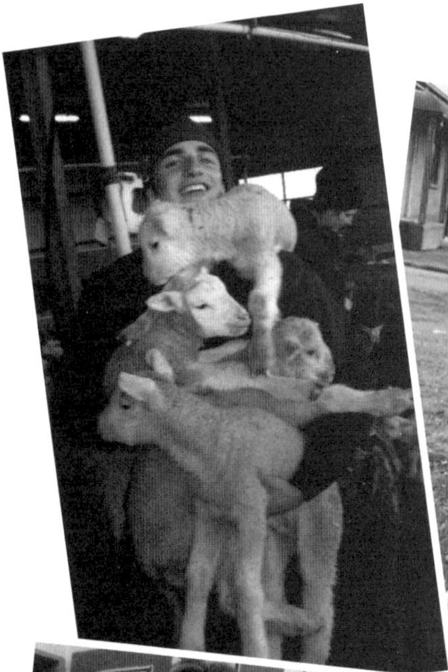

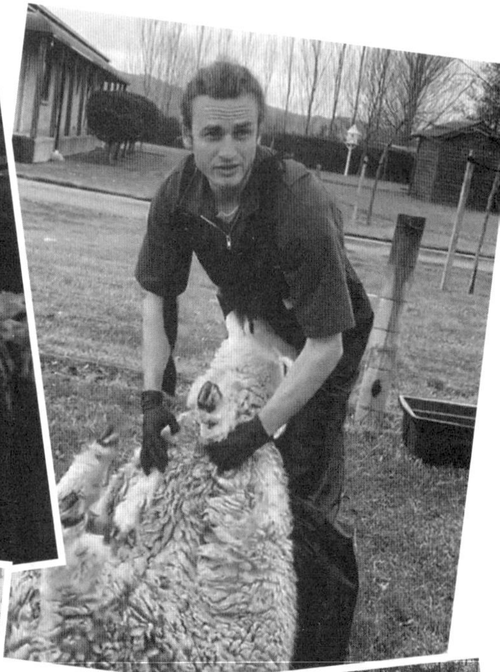

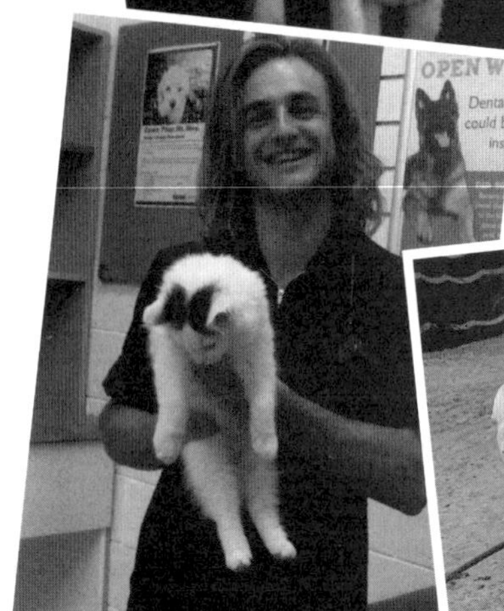
Dental

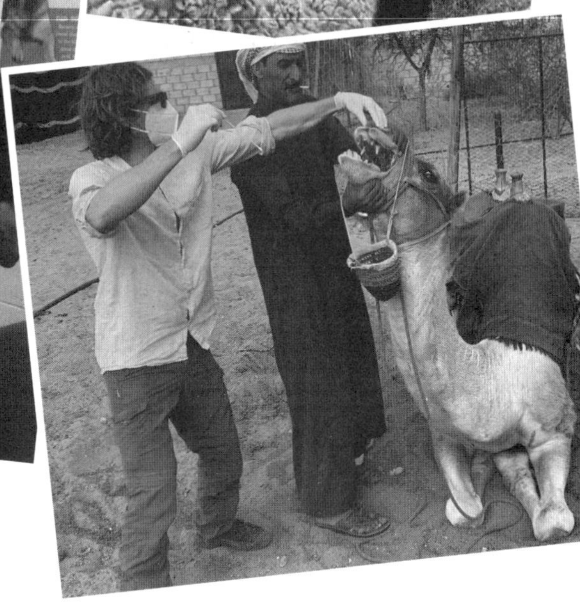

ABOUT THE AUTHOR

MARCUS TAYLOR graduated with a degree in veterinary science from Massey University in 2013 and went straight into mixed practice. He later worked in Newfoundland and southern England, and then he worked for a year on an animal-health research project with the Bedouin in the Middle East. He has run a podcast with a veterinary colleague, and has a YouTube channel, *Lord of the Vets*. He lives in Christchurch, where he works as a writer and veterinary contractor.

MASSEY
UNIVERSITY
PRESS

First published in 2024 by Massey University Press

Private Bag 102904, North Shore Mail Centre
Auckland 0745, New Zealand

www.masseypress.ac.nz

Design: Sarah Elworthy

Cover photograph: Marcus Taylor with Albi the dog,
photo courtesy of the author

Back cover photographs: courtesy of the author

This publication is designed for entertainment purposes only. This book is not intended to be a substitute for the medical advice of a licensed veterinarian. Readers should always consult their veterinarians regarding their animals' health. Neither the publisher nor the author shall be liable for any medical damages, including but not limited to special, incidental, consequential, personal or other damages for any attempts to replicate the methods or activities described in this book.

A catalogue record for this book is available from the National Library of New Zealand

Printed and bound in China by Everbest Printing Investment Limited

ISBN: 978-1-99-101699-7

eISBN: 978-1-99-101689-8